T0294441

Gender Affirming Surgery

Editor

RUSSELL E. ETTINGER

ORAL AND MAXILLOFACIAL SURGERY CLINICS OF NORTH AMERICA

www.oralmaxsurgery.theclinics.com

Consulting Editor
RUI P. FERNANDES

May 2024 • Volume 36 • Number 2

ELSEVIER

1600 John F. Kennedy Boulevard • Suite 1800 • Philadelphia, Pennsylvania, 19103-2899

http://www.oralmaxsurgery.theclinics.com

ORAL AND MAXILLOFACIAL SURGERY CLINICS OF NORTH AMERICA Volume 36, Number 2
May 2024 ISSN 1042-3699, ISBN-13: 978-0-443-12887-5

Editor: John Vassallo; j.vassallo@elsevier.com
Developmental Editor: Anita Chamoli

Oral and Maxillofacial Surgery Clinics of North America (ISSN 1042-3699) is published quarterly by Elsevier Inc., 360 Park Avenue South, New York, NY 10010-1710. Months of issue are February, May, August, and November. Business and Editorial Offices: 1600 John F. Kennedy Blvd., Suite 1800, Philadelphia, PA 19103-2899. Periodicals postage paid at New York, NY and additional mailing offices. Subscription prices are $417.00 per year for US individuals, $100.00 per year for US students/residents, $488.00 per year for Canadian individuals, $100.00 per year for Canadian students/residents, $540.00 per year for international individuals, $235.00 per year for international students/residents. For institutional access pricing please contact Customer Service via the contact information below. To receive student/resident rate, orders must be accompanied by name or affiliated institution, date of term, and the *signature* of program/residency coordinator on institution letterhead. Orders will be billed at individual rate until proof of status is received. Foreign air speed delivery is included in all *Clinics* subscription prices. All prices are subject to change without notice. **POSTMASTER:** Send address changes to *Oral and Maxillofacial Surgery Clinics of North America*, Elsevier Periodicals **Customer Service, 11830 Westline Industrial Drive, St. Louis, MO 63146. Tel: 1-800-654-2452 (U.S. and Canada); 314-447-8871 (outside U.S. and Canada). Fax: 314-447-8029. E-mail: journalscustomerservice-usa@elsevier.com (for print support); journalsonlinesupport-usa@elsevier.com (for online support).**

Reprints. For copies of 100 or more, of articles in this publication, please contact the Commercial Reprints Department, Elsevier Inc., 360 Park Avenue South, New York, NY 10010-1710. Tel.: 212-633-3874; Fax: 212-633-3820; Email: reprints@elsevier.com.

Oral and Maxillofacial Surgery Clinics of North America is covered in *MEDLINE/PubMed (Index Medicus)*, *Science Citation Index Expanded (SciSearch®)*, *Journal Citation Reports/Science Edition*, and *Current Contents®/Clinical Medicine*.

Contributors

CONSULTING EDITOR

RUI P. FERNANDES, MD, DMD, FACS, FRCS(Ed)
Clinical Professor and Chief, Division of Head and Neck Surgery, Program Director, Head and Neck Oncologic Surgery and Microvascular Reconstruction Fellowship,
Departments of Oral and Maxillofacial Surgery, Neurosurgery, and Orthopaedic Surgery and Rehabilitation, University of Florida Health Science Center, University of Florida College of Medicine, Jacksonville, Florida

EDITOR

RUSSELL E. ETTINGER, MD
Assistant Professor, Section of Plastic and Reconstructive Surgery, Division of Plastic Surgery, Department of Surgery, University of Washington; Assistant Professor, Harborview
Medical Center, Division of Craniofacial and Plastic Surgery, Department of Surgery, Seattle Children's Hospital, Seattle, Washington

AUTHORS

ARYA ANDRE AKHAVAN, MD
Plastic Surgery Resident, Division of Plastic and Reconstructive Surgery, Rutgers New Jersey Medical School, Newark, New Jersey; Director of Research, Align Surgical Associates, San Francisco, California

MONA ASCHA, MD
Fellow, Department of Plastic and Reconstructive Surgery, Center for Transgender and Gender Expansive Health, Johns Hopkins Hospital, Baltimore, Maryland

THAIS CALDERON, MD
Resident Physician, Division of Plastic Surgery, Department of Surgery, University of Washington Medical Center, Seattle, Washington

BRENDAN J. CRONIN, MD
Resident Physician, Division of Plastic and Reconstructive Surgery, University of California, Los Angeles, Los Angeles, California

DANIELLE EBLE, MD
Resident Physician, Division of Plastic Surgery, Department of Surgery, University of Washington, Seattle, Washington

RUSSELL E. ETTINGER, MD
Assistant Professor, Section of Plastic and Reconstructive Surgery, Division of Plastic Surgery, Department of Surgery, University of Washington; Assistant Professor, Harborview Medical Center, Division of Craniofacial and Plastic Surgery, Department of Surgery, Seattle Children's Hospital, Seattle, Washington

MATTHEW GOLDENBERG, PsyD
Psychologist, Gender Clinic, Adolescent Medicine Seattle Children's Hospital, Seattle, Washington

BASHAR HASSAN, MD
Postdoctoral Research Fellow, Department of Plastic and Reconstructive Surgery, Center for Transgender and Gender Expansive Health, Johns Hopkins Hospital, Baltimore, Maryland

CORINNE S. HEINEN, MD
Clinical Professor, Family Medicine and
Internal Medicine, Division of Allergy and
Infectious Disease, University of Washington,
Harborview Medical Center, Seattle,
Washington

EMILY HEM
Patient Care Coordinator, Division of Plastic
Surgery, Department of Surgery, University of
Washington, Seattle, Washington

WILLIAM Y. HOFFMAN, MD
Professor of Surgery, Division of Plastic and
Reconstructive Surgery, University of
California San Francisco, San Francisco,
California

SEAN L. JOHNSON, LSWAIC
Program Director of Transgender and Gender
Non-Binary Health Program, Office of
Healthcare Equity, University of Washington
School of Medicine, Seattle, Washington

CORAL KATAVE, BA
Third Year Medical Student, Pre-doctoral
Research Fellow, Division of Plastic and
Reconstructive Surgery, Brigham and
Women's Hospital, Harvard Medical School,
Boston, Massachusetts

JACQUELYN KNOX, MD
Plastic Surgery Resident, Division of Plastic
and Reconstructive Surgery, University of
California San Francisco, San Francisco,
California

JUSTINE C. LEE, MD, PhD
Professor and Associate Chief, Division of
Plastic and Reconstructive Surgery, University
of California, Los Angeles, Los Angeles,
California

FAN LIANG, MD
Assistant Professor, Department of Plastic and
Reconstructive Surgery, Center for
Transgender and Gender Expansive Health,
Johns Hopkins Hospital, Baltimore, Maryland

SHANE D. MORRISON, MD
Surgeon, Division of Plastic Surgery,
Department of Surgery, University of
Washington School of Medicine, University of
Washington, Seattle, Washington

JOHN HENRY PANG, MD
Surgeon, Align Surgical Associates, San
Francisco, California

ELIE P. RAMLY, MD
Plastic and Reconstructive Surgery Resident,
Harvard Medical School, Brigham and
Women's Hospital, Boston, Massachusetts

KAVITHA RANGANATHAN, MD
Director of Craniofacial Reconstruction,
Assistant Professor of Surgery, Division of
Plastic and Reconstructive Surgery, Brigham
and Women's Hospital, Harvard Medical
School, Boston, Massachusetts

THOMAS SATTERWHITE, MD
CEO and Surgeon, Align Surgical Associates,
San Francisco, California; Adjunct Clinical
Assistant Professor, Division of Plastic and
Reconstructive Surgery, Department of
Surgery, Stanford University Medical Center,
Palo Alto, California

SRINIVAS SUSARLA, DMD, MD, MPH
Associate Professor, Division of Plastic
Surgery, Department of Surgery, University of
Washington; Harborview Medical Center,
Division of Craniofacial and Plastic Surgery,
Department of Surgery, Seattle Children's
Hospital, Seattle, Washington

PHIL TOLLEY, MD
Resident, Division of Plastic Surgery,
Department of Surgery, University of
Washington, Harborview Medical Center,
Seattle, Washington

TANNON L. TOPLE, BS
Medical Student, Department of Medicine,
University of Minnesota Twin Cities Medical
School, Minneapolis, Minnesota

Contents

Preface: Gender-Affirming Facial Surgery ix

Russell E. Ettinger

Epidemiology of Gender Diversity 137

Tannon L. Tople, Thais Calderon, and Sean L. Johnson

In the United States, approximately 1.6 million individuals identify as transgender and gender diverse (TGD), encompassing a wide range of identities and experiences. Despite progress in visibility and acceptance, TGD people continue to face health care and societal disparities, especially affecting racial minorities. Although legal advancements have been achieved, the key to addressing these persistent health care disparities lies in implementing comprehensive and culturally sensitive health care practices and supportive policies. With a growing number of TGD people seeking gender-affirming care, it is imperative that health care practitioners understand the unique challenges faced by this community and provide tailored services with sensitivity and expertise.

Addressing the Mental Health Needs of Transgender and Gender Diverse Adult Patients Seeking Facial Surgery 143

Matthew Goldenberg

Transgender and gender diverse (TGD) patients may present to a surgical context with complex mental health challenges, many of which stem from external stressors. TGD patients also may face disparities regarding the accessibility and quality of health care experiences, which also erodes the mental health of patients. Providers who offer gender-affirming surgery need to be aware of the context that patients may arrive in and install practices that can address the needs of TGD patients.

Medical Management of Gender Diversity 151

Corinne S. Heinen

This article provides context on the experiences and medical care of individuals who experience gender dysphoria for the benefit of oral and maxillofacial surgeons. The mechanism of action, effects, and side effects of medical therapies used for gender-affirming care are reviewed. Specific guidance for anesthetic care is given. Trauma-informed tools for care of transgender and gender-diverse patients are offered.

Surgical Standards of Care and Insurance Authorization of Gender-Affirming Facial Surgery 161

Danielle Eble and Emily Hem

Transgender and gender-diverse patients face complex, multifactorial barriers to medically necessary gender-affirming care. Insurance coverage for facial feminizing and masculinizing surgeries is one such obstacle. Providers and affiliated team members must have a comprehensive understanding of clinical standards of care, medical documentation, insurance policy and terminology, and related legislation to successfully navigate this administrative quagmire and ensure patient access to care..

Preoperative Radiology and Virtual Surgical Planning   171

Brendan J. Cronin and Justine C. Lee

> Virtual surgical planning enables precise surgical planning and translation of this planning into the operating room. Preoperative maxillofacial computed tomography scans are compared to a reference skull to identify desired surgical changes. In facial feminization surgery, these include forehead recontouring/frontal table setback, gonial angle reduction, and possible chin repositioning/reshaping, while in facial masculinization surgery, this includes forehead augmentation and gonial angle/chin augmentation. Cutting and recontouring guides as well as custom implants are then custom manufactured. Common guides include osteotomy guides, depth drilling guides, ostectomy guides, and guides for one/two-piece genioplasty or chin burring. Common implants include mandibular and chin implants.

Facial Feminization: Upper Third of the Face   183

Elie P. Ramly, Coral Katave, and Kavitha Ranganathan

> Facial feminization surgery (FFS) is a crucial intervention for transgender women. This article delves into comprehensive reconstruction of the upper third of the face, discussing anatomic differences between masculine and feminine features, and surgical considerations. Technical considerations, preoperative planning, procedural approaches, and postoperative care are described in detail. Patient-centered operative planning and execution ensure safety and efficacy in FFS and uphold its transformative effect on quality of life in appropriately selected surgical candidates.

Facial Feminization: Middle Third of the Face   195

Mona Ascha, Bashar Hassan, and Fan Liang

> Facial feminization surgery (FFS) as applied to the midfacial region targets modifications to the nasal and malar esthetic complexes. Although a global assessment is paramount in achieving desired functional results, most patients benefit from malar feminization in the form of bony and soft tissue augmentation, and nasal feminization in the form of reductive rhinoplasty. For patients with signs of aging, additional interventions in the form of rhytidectomy are powerful adjuncts to feminization. As with FFS techniques directed toward the upper and lower thirds, the overarching goal is to obtain complementary outcomes that enhance facial harmony and beauty.

Gender-Affirming Facial Surgery: Lower Third of the Face   207

Phil Tolley, Srinivas Susarla, and Russell E. Ettinger

> This article is intended to give the reader an overview of facial gender-affirming procedures applicable to the lower face and neck. A review of facial analysis in the context of masculine versus feminine facial features and the contributions of both soft tissue and bone to this anatomy is provided. The use of systematic facial evaluation and patient-driven concerns as a guide for presurgical planning is reviewed. Detailed descriptions of the unique surgical interventions to feminize the soft tissues and the skeletal framework of the lower face and neck are provided.

Gender Affirming Facial Surgery–Anatomy and Procedures for Facial Masculinization   221

Arya Andre Akhavan, John Henry Pang, Shane D. Morrison, and Thomas Satterwhite

For some patients, feminine facial features may cause significant gender dysphoria. Multiple nonsurgical and surgical techniques exist to masculinize facial features. Nonsurgical techniques include testosterone supplementation and dermal fillers. Surgical techniques include soft tissue manipulation, synthetic implants, regenerative scaffolding, or bony reconstruction. Many techniques are derived from experience with cisgender patients, but are adapted with special considerations to differing anatomy between cisgender and transgender men and women. Currently, facial masculinization is less commonly sought than feminization, but demand is likely to increase as techniques are refined and made available.

Facial Gender-Affirming Surgery: Pitfalls, Complications, and How to Avoid Them   237

Jacquelyn Knox and William Y. Hoffman

Facial feminization is a complex undertaking requiring skill in both craniofacial and aesthetic plastic surgery. As in aesthetic procedures, understanding the patient's goals and setting realistic expectations in light of an individual's anatomy is critical. Both soft tissue and bone must be addressed to adequately soften masculine facial features. This article delves into specific anatomic areas and delineates some of the pathways to successful outcomes.

ORAL AND MAXILLOFACIAL SURGERY CLINICS OF NORTH AMERICA

FORTHCOMING ISSUES

August 2024
Pediatric Craniomaxillofacial Pathology
Srinivas M. Susarla, *Editor*

November 2024
Perforator Flaps for Head and Neck Reconstruction
Susana Heredero, *Editor*

February 2025
Long Term Outcomes in Implant Dentistry
Nardy Casap and Michael Alterman, *Editors*

RECENT ISSUES

February 2024
Molecular, Therapeutic, and Surgical Updates on Head and Neck Vascular Anomalies
Srinivasa Rama Chandra and Sanjiv Nair, *Editors*

November 2023
Pediatric Craniomaxillofacial Trauma
Srinivas M. Susarla, *Editor*

August 2023
Imaging of Common Oral Cavity, Sinonasal, and Skull Base Pathology
Dinesh Rao, *Editor*

SERIES OF RELATED INTEREST

Atlas of the Oral and Maxillofacial Surgery Clinics
www.oralmaxsurgeryatlas.theclinics.com

Dental Clinics
www.dental.theclinics.com

THE CLINICS ARE NOW AVAILABLE ONLINE!
Access your subscription at:
www.theclinics.com

Preface
Gender-Affirming Facial Surgery

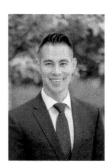

Russell E. Ettinger, MD
Editor

The face is inherently the most visible and arguably the most socially significant component of an individual's identity. Our facial form is how we represent ourselves to the external world and shapes how we progress through it. As a social species, humans have survived and thrived based on our ability to interact with those around us and form close-knit societal groups. Complex facial expression and our ability to decern the minutia of subtle facial ques were integral to our survival advantage and have been slowly perfected over millennia. The evolutionary importance of the facial form to primate species extends to the cellular level where single neurons within the visual cortex, termed "face neurons," are known to fully activate only when presented with an image of a face. Consequently, all humans, whether we appreciate it or not, are experts in deciphering facial forms and determining which elements align and those that do not.

As facial surgeons, we are charged with the responsibility to modify, enhance, and restore the form and function of the face to not only improve health but also allow our patients to present to the outside world and move through society without stigma or discrimination. Gender-affirming facial surgery represents a culmination of techniques and lessons learned from the pioneering craniofacial, oral maxillofacial, and head and neck surgeons who shaped our individual subspecialities. Facial gender-affirming surgery borrows concepts from trauma surgery, aesthetic surgery, and reconstructive surgery alike and offers a path for individuals to align their physical appearance with their internal sense of self.

Holistic care for gender-diverse individuals is predicated on close collaboration between numerous heath care providers of various backgrounds outside of surgery. As such, we are fortunate in this issue to have a diverse compendium of authors who are experts within their respective fields of gender-affirming health care. Through the lens of their expertise, we hope to provide the readership with a broad understanding of gender diversity and the specific challenges that gender-diverse individuals face on their journey to authentic self-expression. With that common understanding, we can then better frame the impact of gender-affirming facial surgery as we delve into care models, insurance-approval processes, preoperative planning, and the surgical techniques and pitfalls of facial feminization and

Oral Maxillofacial Surg Clin N Am 36 (2024) ix–x
https://doi.org/10.1016/j.coms.2024.02.002
1042-3699/24/

masculinization procedures. I am eternally grateful to all of our contributing authors, who have extended us time from their personal and professional lives to enhance our understanding of a complex topic. I would also like to express my gratitude to the editorial staff at the *Oral and Maxillofacial Surgery Clinics of North America*, specifically, John Vassallo and Anita Chamoli, for their guidance and diligence on the production of a yet another high-yield issue for the readership. Finally, I would like to thank my wife and children for their unconditional love and support through my years of training and active surgical practice.

Russell E. Ettinger, MD
Department of Surgery
University of Washington
Section of Plastic and Reconstructive Surgery
Harborview Medical Center
325 9th Avenue
Seattle, WA 98104, USA

Epidemiology of Gender Diversity

Tannon L. Tople, BS[a],*, Thais Calderon, MD[b], Sean L. Johnson, LSWAIC[c,1]

KEYWORDS

- Transgender • Gender identity • Gender-affirming care • Gender diversity epidemiology
- Gender-affirming surgery • Facial feminization surgery

KEY POINTS

- The transgender and gender diverse (TGD) population in the United States includes a significant number of people encompassing transgender, nonbinary, and gender diverse identities.
- TGD people face substantial disparities in health, socioeconomic status, and access to gender-affirming care, with marked differences across racial and ethnic groups.
- Legal and policy developments, such as the Affordable Care Act's Section 1557, have improved access to gender-affirming treatments, yet barriers and disparities persist.
- Increased visibility and societal acceptance of TGD identities primarily account for the growing number of TGD people observed in recent decades.

DEFINITIONS/BACKGROUND

Transgender is a term that describes a person's gender identity that differs from the sex assigned to them at birth. Although the term transgender includes nonbinary and gender-diverse identities broadly, these latter terms describe gender identities that may not conform to traditional gender binaries (eg, masculine vs feminine), encompass multiple genders or have no gender. On the other hand, gender identity refers to one's innate sense of gender. Transitioning refers to the process in which a person begins living in their gender that is different from the one assigned to them on their birth certificate. Intersectionality is a term used to describe the interconnection between social identities such as race, gender, and socioeconomic status applied to an individual or given group and emphasize overlapping systems of discrimination. As gender is socially constructed and changing over time and across cultures, self-identification and expression of gender within the transgender and gender diverse (TGD) population vary greatly.

Similarly, gender-affirming surgical and medical care needs vary within this population, as does access to this care across the United States, with inclusive and knowledgeable health care practitioners being needed by all.

EPIDEMIOLOGY OF GENDER DIVERSITY

An estimated 1.6 million people (0.39%–2.7%) in the United States identify as TGD, though the true population of TGD people remains difficult to quantify.[1–5] Within this community, 33% identify as transgender women, 29% as transgender men, and 35% as nonbinary persons,[6] with almost half of all transgender adults (transgender men: 47%; transgender women: 46%) being 25 to 44 years of age. Nonbinary people are more likely to be younger, with 61% being aged 18 to 24, compared with 43% and 24% of transgender men and women in the same age group, respectively.[6] Transitioning also happens relatively early in life, with the majority (43%) of people beginning

[a] Department of Medicine, University of Minnesota Twin Cities Medical School, 420 Delaware Street Southeast, Minneapolis, MN 55455, USA; [b] Division of Plastic Surgery, Department of Surgery, University of Washington Medical Center, 325 9th Avenue, Box 359796, Seattle, WA 98104, USA; [c] Office of Healthcare Equity, University of Washington School of Medicine, 1959 Northeast Pacific Street, F-Wing, Seattle, WA, USA
[1] Present address: 4333 Brooklyn Avenue Northeast, Seattle, WA 98105.
* Corresponding author.
E-mail address: tople004@umn.edu

Oral Maxillofacial Surg Clin N Am 36 (2024) 137–142
https://doi.org/10.1016/j.coms.2023.12.003
1042-3699/24/© 2023 Elsevier Inc. All rights reserved.

this process between 18 and 24 years of age; however, the recognition of one's innate gender identity occurs at even earlier ages, with 83% of people recognizing they are transgender between ages 5 and 20 years.[6] As more people begin identifying as TGD and transitioning at younger ages, the demographics of future TGD populations may be expected to change.[7]

Racial identities of TGD people in the United States provide critical insight into the diverse composition of this community. According to the US Transgender Survey (USTS) conducted in 2015 and considered the most extensive dataset on TGD people available at the time of writing this article, the racial and ethnic distribution of the respondents varied. The survey reported that 62.2% identified as White, 12.6% as African American or Black, 16.6% as Latinx, and 5.1% as Asian.[6] Although White TGD people were overrepresented in this sample, the diversity depicted in the survey reflects the intersectionality within the community, where racial identities and corresponding gender identities shape individual experiences and challenges. The disparities in health care access, social acceptance, and economic opportunities often vary significantly across these racial and ethnic groups, revealing a complex landscape that requires nuanced understanding and tailored approaches to address the specific needs and issues faced within the TGD community.

The visibility of the TGD community has also continued to grow in the past decade. According to the USTS, the response rate from TGD people in 2015 was four times higher than in the previous 2008 to 2009 survey.[6] Increased visibility and societal acceptance of TGD identities primarily account for the growing number of TGD people observed in recent decades, as estimates suggest that the community's true size has actually remained steady over time.[5,8,9] Efforts to identify TGD people are also growing, contributing to the noticeable increase in TGD people. For example, in 2016, the Centers for Medicare and Medicaid Services required that sexual orientation and gender identity (SOGI) questions be available in electronic health records.[10] This effort has improved the reporting of SOGI in health records and made advances to population-based surveys. In addition, an increase in state-based inclusive policy developments has aided efforts to identify TGD people. Changes to state and federal identification documents, such as allowing more people to identify outside of the gender binary on their driver's license, have contributed to the noticeable recorded increase of TGD people.[11] As improvements in identifying TGD people continue to be

expected, it is essential to recognize the TGD community as a patient population that is growing in salience and requiring distinct care throughout the United States.

The proportion of transgender men to women has been a subject of discussion. Historically, studies have reported differing ratios, with some indicating a higher number of transgender women compared with transgender men, a reverse of this ratio, or an even distribution.[12] These discrepancies are likely attributable to differences in study methodologies, geographic locations, cultural contexts, and definitions of gender categories. For example, a study by Meerwijk and Sevelius noted that the ratio of transgender women to men varied widely across different countries, reflecting the complex interplay of cultural, social, and economic factors.[8] On the other hand, other studies indicate that the ratio of transgender men to women has remained relatively 1:1,[13,14] with only limited reports of this ratio increasing due to more adolescent boys seeking treatment.[15] In addition to assessing population data for transgender men and women, more notable demographics have been observed in nonbinary adolescents. One state-based population study found that among TGD adolescents, 50% were likely to identify as nonbinary.[16] This research underscores some potentially notable demographics within the TGD community, as nonbinary people are more prevalent among adolescents. Ultimately, understanding the true proportion of TGD people requires careful consideration and suggests a need for standardized research practices in the field.

DISPARITIES IN THE TRANSGENDER AND GENDER DIVERSE COMMUNITY

TGD people experience significant economic, health, and social disparities across many institutions. Economically, the TGD community faces acute challenges. According to data provided by the USTS, more than one-third of the TGD community live below the poverty line, 33% have experienced homelessness, and unemployment rates are triple that of the general US population.[6] Unfortunately, even for those in the workforce, TGD people are less likely to be promoted and more prone to being fired and mistreated compared with their cisgender colleagues.[6] Experiences also differ between age groups. For example, TGD youth face even greater disparities due to family rejection, discrimination, and violence. TGD youth have greater odds of experiencing homelessness and housing instability compared with cisgender LGBQ (Lesbian, Gay, Bisexual, and Queer) youth, with TGD and other LGBQ-identified youth estimated to make up 20% to 40% of 1.6 million homeless youth.[17,18] Taken together, these findings highlight pervasive discrimination that adversely affects the financial stability of TGD people. The resulting socioeconomic vulnerability, in turn, impinges on access to health care resources, engendering a vicious cycle where health disparities also contribute to the overall socioeconomic inequities faced by this community.

Race and TGD identities intersect, leading to increased discrimination. For example, Black, Indigenous, and People of Color TGD people have higher rates of homelessness, are three times more likely to be living under the poverty line (12%), and have four times greater unemployment rates (20%) than the US unemployment rate (5%).[6] Similarly, TGD people of color face higher HIV rates, with Black transgender women contracting the virus at higher frequencies (19%).[6] These examples highlight the growing inequities in socioeconomic status and health, compounded by discrimination against intersecting identities.

Undocumented TGD people and TGD people with disabilities also face severe disparities. Undocumented TGD people face economic hardship, violence, and homelessness, with 50% having been homeless and 68% facing intimate partner violence.[6] In addition, one-quarter of TGD people with disabilities are unemployed, and 45% live in poverty.[6] TGD people with disabilities also reported higher rates of psychological distress (59%) and mistreatment by health care practitioners (42%).[6] These alarming statistics not only shed light on the multidimensional challenges faced by undocumented and TGD individuals with disabilities but also underscore the urgent need for targeted interventions and policies that address them.

The health disparities within the TGD community are further perpetuated through inequities in insurance coverage. Many TGD people encounter significant barriers in accessing health care insurance that is both affordable and comprehensive in the services offered.[19] Studies have found that a substantial proportion of TGD people are either underinsured or completely uninsured, as compared with their cisgender counterparts.[6] These disparities are frequently linked to systemic biases within the insurance industry, leading to the exclusion of critical gender-affirming treatments and procedures from coverage. For example, 25% and 55% of TGD people seeking hormonal therapy and gender-affirming surgery (GAS) were denied coverage, respectively.[6]

For those unable to get their care covered by insurance, the cost of necessary medical care can also be prohibitively expensive. This can lead to unmet health care needs and further aggravate existing health disparities. Thus, health insurance acts as another barrier for TGD people seeking gender-affirming treatments.

Access to general health care can also be limited by health care systems due to a lack of understanding, empathy, and specialized care toward TGD people among health care practitioners. Even when medical care is available, transgender patients may face unequal treatment, lack of respect, and refusal of gender-affirming care.[6] Approximately, one-third of patients have a negative experience with their health care practitioner, and less than one-quarter will avoid seeing a doctor out of fear of being mistreated.[6] Mistreatment within the medical system frequently results in delays or outright avoidance of medical treatment, contributing to poorer overall health outcomes. Moreover, social stigma and discrimination further contribute to these disparities by exacerbating stress and other mental health challenges. Coordinated efforts must be made to train health care professionals to be culturally competent, reform insurance practices, and promote societal understanding to mitigate these disparities and improve the overall health and well-being of the TGD community.[20]

Discrimination perpetuated by both health care practitioners and insurance has led to overall worse health outcomes for the TGD community. Mental health outcomes, in particular, are poor, with 40% of TGD people having attempted suicide within their lifetime and 39% experiencing severe psychological distress.[6] Such alarming statistics can be linked to the systemic barriers faced by TGD individuals within the health care system, including the denial of coverage for gender-affirming procedures, refusal of care, and the stigmatizing attitudes of some health care practitioners. Access to gender-affirming care and procedures is paramount to improving these health outcomes. One study found that the initiation of gender-affirming care (puberty blockers and gender-affirming hormones) for youth lowered the odds of depression by 60% and suicidality by 73%, whereas another found that the reduction of mental health treatment needed continued to decrease years after GAS.[21] Moreover, the lack of specialized training in transgender health issues among medical professionals further compounds these problems leading to improper treatment or reluctance to seek care altogether. The cumulative effect of these discriminatory practices can significantly hinder access to essential health care services for TGD people, thereby exacerbating mental health issues and worsening quality of life.

TRENDS IN GENDER-AFFIRMING SURGERY

Because the passage of the Affordable Care Act and the incorporation of Section 1557, TGD people have increasingly sought gender-affirming care. Section 1557, which prevents the discrimination of patients based on sex in health care settings, insurance coverage determinations, and insurance eligibility, was officially reinterpreted in 2016 and increased protections for TGD people.[22] This new interpretation expanded protections by prohibiting transgender exclusions in health insurance plans and ensuring that insurers cannot deny coverage of services offered to TGD people that may otherwise be given to cisgender patients.[23] As a result, more TGD people have become insured since 2016, and the utilization of gender-affirming care has risen.[24] In addition, as of 2023, 24 states and the District of Colombia have taken additional measures to prohibit private insurance companies from explicitly refusing to cover transgender health services.[23] Although there has been improvement, coverage of specific GASs continues to be controlled on a state-by-state basis.

Increased legal protections have directly led to increased utilization of gender-affirming services. Between 2015 and 2018, following the reinterpretation of Section 1577, the volume of transfeminine and transmasculine surgeries increased by 109% and 392%, respectively.[24] A granular analysis of these procedures also demonstrated that between 2013 and 2018, there were 13.6 times the number of patients undergoing facial feminization surgeries (FFSs).[25] Although noticeable demand has been seen, these metrics may still underrepresent the current utilization of this care as practitioners learn to code these procedures in the medical record more accurately. Future state legislation changes may also improve or restrict access to GAS, thus impacting the utilization of services. Although some insurance/coverage barriers have been reduced, the surge in surgical requests has highlighted the need for a greater number of skilled surgical practitioners, as well as increased system capacity to provide these services, as wait times can often extend beyond a year or more for most surgical programs.[26] As more states cover procedures, a growing number of health care resources is needed to accommodate the number of TGD people seeking out gender-affirming care.

The frequency of who seeks care has also been investigated. Transgender men and women seem to seek gender-affirming hormonal therapies and surgeries at the same rate, though some differences in the type of surgery sought exist. For example, research conducted by Kaiser Permanente assessed transgender men and women in California and Georgia and their utilization of gender-affirming services. They found that approximately the same proportion of transmasculine and transfeminine patients received hormone therapy and genital surgery, whereas transgender men were more likely to undergo chest surgery (12% vs 0.3%).[13,14] These data indicate that the ratio of transgender men and women seeking care remains relatively equal but also highlights some differences in the need for GAS based on gender identity.

CURRENT RESEARCH ON FACIAL FEMINIZATION SURGERY OUTCOMES

Considerable progress has been made in understanding how GASs improve the lives of TGD people. Specifically, a focus on whether FFS improves the quality of life for TGD patients has been studied. In a 2023 study analyzing 11 patient-reported outcomes, researchers found that patients noted significant improvements among seven psychosocial categories after surgery, such as anxiety, anger, depression, positive affect, meaning and purpose, global mental health, and social isolation.[27] Similarly, a prospective international study of 66 patients found that patients were highly satisfied with their surgery following FFS.[28] Furthermore, identical benefits to patients' quality of life have been observed following gender-affirming mastectomies and genital surgery.[29–31] Findings from both studies emphasize that FFS can improve patients' quality of life, a key finding that supports the use of FFS for treating gender dysphoria.

Some limitations do exist in the data surrounding FFS and patient-reported outcomes. Specifically, there is a paucity of long-term follow-up studies using validated survey instruments assessing FFS outcomes. Completion of these studies is necessary to understand the comprehensive physical, emotional, and social effects of FFS. As existing research tends to have shorter follow-ups assessing outcomes related to FFS, more must be done to expand on current findings.[32]

Overall, encouraging patient-reported outcomes described in the current literature, combined with the growing acceptance and recognition of the importance of GAS, has led to an increase in these procedures. Considering this, it is not surprising that as of 2023, close to one-quarter of TGD people have had some type of GAS.[6] As continued research, policy support, and health care practitioner education efforts are conducted, more TGD people than ever will be seeking gender-affirming care.

CLINICS CARE POINTS

- Gender-affirming care, including hormonal therapy and gender-affirming surgery, improves mental health and overall well-being, but not providing timely access to gender-affirming treatments and surgeries can contribute to mental health challenges.

- The intersectionality of gender, race, and socioeconomic factors influences the individual needs of the transgender and gender diverse (TGD) community, and failing to recognize the diverse identities and experiences within the TGD community can lead to inadequate care.

- Discrimination in the insurance industry remains a significant obstacle, leading to unequal access to gender-affirming treatments and procedures.

- As more TGD people seek gender-affirming care, there is a growing need for skilled practitioners and expanded health care system capacity to accommodate the demand for these services.

DISCLOSURE

The authors have nothing to disclose.

REFERENCES

1. Deutsch MB. Making It Count: Improving Estimates of the Size of Transgender and Gender Nonconforming Populations. LGBT Health 2016;3(3):181–5.
2. Gn R, Bj M, Al G, et al. Health and Care Utilization of Transgender and Gender Nonconforming Youth: A Population-Based Study. Pediatrics 2018;141(3). https://doi.org/10.1542/peds.2017-1683.
3. El M, Jm S. Transgender Population Size in the United States: a Meta-Regression of Population-Based Probability Samples. Am J Public Health 2017;107(2). https://doi.org/10.2105/AJPH.2016.303578.
4. Brown A. About 5% of young adults in the U.S. say their gender is different from their sex assigned at birth. Pew Research Center. Published June 7, 2022. Available at: https://www.pewresearch.org/short-reads/2022/06/07/about-5-of-young-adults-in-the-u-s-say-their-gender-is-different-from-their-sex-assigned-at-birth/. Accessed May 24, 2023.
5. Herman JL, Flores AR, O'Neill KK. How many adults and youth identify as transgender in the United States? The Williams Institute; 2022.
6. James S, Herman J, Rankin S, Keisling M, Mottet L, Anafi M. The Report of the 2015 U.S. Transgender Survey. Published online 2016. Available at: https://ncvc.dspacedirect.org/handle/20.500.11990/1299. Accessed April 9, 2022.
7. Nolan IT, Kuhner CJ, Dy GW. Demographic and temporal trends in transgender identities and gender confirming surgery. Transl Androl Urol 2019;8(3):184–90.
8. Meerwijk EL, Sevelius JM. Transgender Population Size in the United States: a Meta-Regression of Population-Based Probability Samples. Am J Public Health 2017;107(2):e1–8.
9. MacCarthy S, Reisner SL, Nunn A, et al. The Time Is Now: Attention Increases to Transgender Health in the United States but Scientific Knowledge Gaps Remain. LGBT Health 2015;2(4):287–91.
10. 2015 Edition Health Information Technology (Health IT) Certification Criteria, 2015 Edition Base Electronic Health Record (EHR) Definition, and ONC Health IT Certification Program Modifications. Federal Register. Published October 16, 2015. Available at: https://www.federalregister.gov/documents/2015/10/16/2015-25597/2015-edition-health-information-technology-health-it-certification-criteria-2015-edition-base. Accessed June 15, 2023.
11. Movement Advancement Project | Identity Document Laws and Policies. Available at: https://www.lgbtmap.org/equality-maps/identity_documents. Accessed August 4, 2023.
12. Aitken M, Steensma TD, Blanchard R, et al. Evidence for an altered sex ratio in clinic-referred adolescents with gender dysphoria. J Sex Med 2015;12(3):756–63.
13. Quinn VP, Nash R, Hunkeler E, et al. Cohort profile: Study of Transition, Outcomes and Gender (STRONG) to assess health status of transgender people. BMJ Open 2017;7(12):e018121.
14. Leinung MC, Joseph J. Changing Demographics in Transgender Individuals Seeking Hormonal Therapy: Are Trans Women More Common Than Trans Men? Transgender Health 2020;5(4):241–5.
15. Wiepjes CM, Nota NM, de Blok CJM, et al. The Amsterdam Cohort of Gender Dysphoria Study (1972-2015): Trends in Prevalence, Treatment, and Regrets. J Sex Med 2018;15(4):582–90.
16. Rider GN, McMorris BJ, Gower AL, et al. Health and Care Utilization of Transgender and Gender Nonconforming Youth: A Population-Based Study. Pediatrics 2018;141(3):e20171683.
17. Housing & Homelessness. National Center for Transgender Equality. Published April 22, 2021. Available at: https://transequality.org/issues/housing-homelessness. Accessed August 4, 2023.
18. Homelessness and Housing Instability Among LGBTQ Youth. The Trevor Project. Published February 3, 2022. Available at: https://www.thetrevorproject.org/research-briefs/homelessness-and-housing-instability-among-lgbtq-youth-feb-2022/. Accessed August 4, 2023.

19. Sineath RC, Woodyatt C, Sanchez T, et al. Determinants of and Barriers to Hormonal and Surgical Treatment Receipt Among Transgender People. Transgender Health 2016;1(1):129–36.

20. Deutsch MB. Guidelines for the Primary and Gender-Affirming Care of Transgender and Gender Nonbinary People. Published 2016. Available at: https://transcare.ucsf.edu/guidelines/breast-cancer-men. Accessed April 9, 2022.

21. Tordoff DM, Wanta JW, Collin A, et al. Mental Health Outcomes in Transgender and Nonbinary Youths Receiving Gender-Affirming Care. JAMA Netw Open 2022;5(2):e220978.

22. 45 CFR Part 92 – Nondiscrimination on the Basis of Race, Color, National Origin, Sex, Age, or Disability in Health Programs or Activities Receiving Federal Financial Assistance and Programs or Activities Administered by the Department of Health and Human Services Under Title I of the Patient Protection and Affordable Care Act or by Entities Established Under Such Title. Available at: https://www.ecfr.gov/current/title-45/part-92. Accessed July 31, 2023.

23. Nondiscrimination in Health Programs and Activities. Federal Register. Published May 18, 2016. Available at: https://www.federalregister.gov/documents/2016/05/18/2016-11458/nondiscrimination-in-health-programs-and-activities. Accessed June 15, 2023.

24. Wiegmann AL, Young EI, Baker KE, et al. The Affordable Care Act and Its Impact on Plastic and Gender-Affirmation Surgery. Plast Reconstr Surg 2021;147(1):135e.

25. Chaya BF, Berman ZP, Boczar D, et al. Current Trends in Facial Feminization Surgery: An Assessment of Safety and Style. J Craniofac Surg 2021;32(7):2366–9.

26. Smith JR, Pakvasa M, Oostrom LA, et al. Transgender gender-affirming surgery consultation among patients seeking care in the Midwestern United States. Medicine (Baltim) 2022;101(45): e31319.

27. Caprini RM, Oberoi MK, Dejam D, et al. Effect of Gender-affirming Facial Feminization Surgery on Psychosocial Outcomes. Ann Surg 2023;277(5): e1184.

28. Morrison SD, Capitán-Cañadas F, Sánchez-García A, et al. Prospective Quality-of-Life Outcomes after Facial Feminization Surgery: An International Multicenter Study. Plast Reconstr Surg 2020;145(6): 1499–509.

29. Branstrom R, Pachankis J. Reduction in Mental Health Treatment Utilization Among Transgender Individuals After Gender-Affirming Surgeries: A Total Population Study. Am J Psychiatry 2019;177(8): 727–34.

30. Lane M, Kirsch MJ, Sluiter EC, et al. Gender Affirming Mastectomy Improves Quality of Life in Transmasculine Patients: A Single-Center Prospective Study. Ann Surg 2021. https://doi.org/10.1097/SLA.0000000000005158.

31. Coleman E, Radix AE, Bouman WP, et al. Standards of Care for the Health of Transgender and Gender Diverse People, Version 8. Int J Transgender Health 2022;23(sup1):S1–259.

32. Morrison SD, Vyas KS, Motakef S, et al. Facial Feminization: Systematic Review of the Literature. Plast Reconstr Surg 2016;137(6):1759–70.

Addressing the Mental Health Needs of Transgender and Gender Diverse Adult Patients Seeking Facial Surgery

Matthew Goldenberg, PsyD

KEYWORDS

- Transgender • Gender diverse • Facial surgery • Mental health needs • Gender-affirming care

KEY POINTS

- Providers should become familiar with the minority stress health model as a foundational concept to address the mental health needs of transgender and gender diverse (TGD) patients.
- Transgender and gender diverse patients face a variety of systemic and interpersonal barriers to accessible and quality health care.
- Providers should become familiar with the standards of care as described by the World Professional Association for Transgender Health.
- Surgical clinics can use a variety of techniques to better invite TGD patients into care.

INTRODUCTION

Transgender and gender diverse (TGD) individuals are a diverse population of individuals who experience incongruence between their gender identity and sex assigned at birth. Gender-affirming care broadly refers to a model of care that assumes gender diversity is a healthy and normal expression of human diversity and that gender itself is not a binary (male or female only) binary. In addition, gender-affirming care assumes that cultures have variation of gender presentations and gender rules, therefore practitioners who seek to work in a gender affirmative manner should exercise cultural sensitivity regarding all individuals. In the gender affirmative model, gender includes biology, development, and socialization as well as specific cultural contexts the individual is exposed to, meaning that gender is a complex phenomenon and cannot be deduced to genitals, personal identity, or any other single factor.[1] The American Medical Association, the American Psychological Association, the American Psychiatric Association, and the American Academy of Pediatrics all endorse gender affirmative care as the most appropriate approach to meet the needs of gender diverse individuals.

The purpose of this article is to examine the mental health needs of gender diverse patients who are seeking facial surgery. There are limited data on the long-term health outcome for transgender adults who receive gender-affirming surgery. However, a meta-analysis of earlier studies completed in 2022 suggests that patients report overwhelmingly positive outcomes after surgery.[2] Attending to the mental health needs of transgender patients can further improve the outcomes for patients who receive gender-affirming surgery.

Of note, there is ample opportunity to expand on the current body of research pertaining to the mental health needs of TGD patients, especially for patients who are seeking service in a surgical context. Although the gender affirmative model makes clear that gender diversity itself is not

Seattle Children's Hospital, Adolescent Medicine, Gender Clinic, 4540 Sand Point Way NE, Seattle, WA 98105, USA
E-mail address: matt.goldenberg@seattlechildrens.org

Oral Maxillofacial Surg Clin N Am 36 (2024) 143–149
https://doi.org/10.1016/j.coms.2023.12.001

pathologic, the increasing marginalization and discrimination that gender diverse individuals face creates outsized mental health disparities within the community. A useful model to begin to conceptualize the mental health effects of chronic systemic and interpersonal challenges for gender diverse patients is the minority stress health model as proposed by Hendricks and Testa.[3] The minority stress health model includes examination of external factors such as higher rate of physical violence, sexual violence, and widespread discrimination, which serves as correlation for negative health outcomes. In a large sample study of more than 27,000 transgender Americans completed in 2015, 47% of respondents reported they had been sexually assaulted at some point in their lifetime, whereas 54% reported some form of intimate partner violence.[4] In terms of discrimination, transgender individuals living in the United States are currently experiencing a barrage of anti-transgender legislation which seeks to limit access to health care, education, public accommodations, inclusion in sports, and ability to change identity documents. The health implications for TGD people who face widescale discrimination are serious and contribute to internal factors of minority stress such as the expectation of violence.[3]

The effect of increased internal and external markers of stress likely contributes to a suicide attempt rate in the TGD population which is nearly five times higher than the general population, whereas the estimated rate for completed suicide is 19 times higher for TGD people than the general population.[5] TGD patients who have a history of depression or substance abuse are at additional risk of attempting suicide; thus, providers caring for TGD patients should include a brief history of mental and psychiatric care history in the standard intake or consultation.[6]

LACK OF TRAINING IN PROVIDERS

A contributing factor in assessing the mental health needs of TGD patients is that few medical providers have had effective training to meet the needs of their patients; hence, providers largely report a lack of knowledge in working with TGD patients.[7] The expected lack of training in medical providers likely contributes to the stress of TGD patients who are seeking medical care. For instance, a 2011 study survey of 132 medical schools in the United States found the median time of training medical students in working with lesbian, gay, bisexual, and transgender patients is 5 hours.[8] Surgical providers likely have had less education on plastic surgery in-service examinations for patients seeking gender-affirming

care.[9] There is significant stress for TGD patients who may feel burdened to continue to work with health care providers who are not well trained due to the scarcity of experienced providers. TGD patients may also struggle to be forthcoming regarding their current needs or medical history with providers they perceive to be unable to provide effective care.

In addition to the risk of being met with a health care provider who has limited knowledge of gender-affirming care needs, patients have reported that providers can express unhelpful behaviors such as using the wrong name in addressing the patient and withholding information.[10] Any patient whose provider does not correctly address them by name and pronoun may experience initial confusion and may have trouble trusting the advice and counsel from medical providers, but TGD patients may also experience misnaming or misgendering as a microaggression and not as a momentary mistake. Additional studies have found that patients may be subject to outright denial of medical care based on their transgender status.[11] In the US Trans survey, 33% of respondents reported having at least one negative experience with a health care provider related to being transgender in the prior year.[4] Negative experiences included being refused treatment, verbally harassed, or physically or sexually assaulted, or having to teach the provider about transgender people to receive appropriate care.

Importantly, potential denial of care is not limited to the direct medical provider and could include administrative clinic staff, pharmacists, patient navigators, and other professionals who represent the patient's broader health care team. In addition to potential denial of care, each member of the staff representative of the surgical and medical team should be cognizant to use the chosen name, pronoun, and prefix of the patient to ensure the patient is receiving care equitable to care provided to cisgender or non-TGD patients. Further, written documentation including chart notes, after visit summaries, and communications with other providers should reflect, whenever possible, the chosen name, pronoun, and prefix of the patient. Patient facing materials such as the name and pronoun written down in the treatment room as well as the personal identification wristband should also reflect the chosen name and pronoun.[12]

WORLD PROFESSIONAL ASSOCIATION FOR TRANSGENDER HEALTH GUIDELINES

The World Professional Association for Transgender Health (WPATH), now in its 8th version, offers flexible guidelines which inform standards of care for transgender youth and adults. Following is the statement of recommendations published by the WPATH which details recommended criteria for transgender patients seeking surgery.[13]

- Gender diversity/incongruence is marked and sustained over time.
- Meets the diagnostic criteria of gender incongruence in situations where a diagnosis is necessary to access health care.
- Demonstrates the emotional and cognitive maturity required to provide informed consent/assent for the treatment.
- Mental health concerns (if any) that may interfere with diagnostic clarity, capacity to consent, and gender-affirming medical treatments have been addressed, sufficiently so that gender-affirming medical treatment can be provided optimally.
- Informed of the reproductive effects, including the potential loss of fertility and the available options to preserve fertility.
- At least 12 months of gender-affirming hormone therapy or longer, if required, to achieve the desired surgical result for gender-affirming procedures, including breast augmentation, orchiectomy, vaginoplasty, hysterectomy, phalloplasty, metoidioplasty, and facial surgery as part of gender-affirming treatment unless hormone therapy is either not desired or is medically contraindicated.

Previous versions of the standards of care recommended a letter of referral from a licensed mental health provider be submitted as part of the surgical referral. In standards of care version 8, a recommendation for written documentation is not explicit, however, "if written documentation or a letter is required to recommend gender-affirming medical and surgical treatment, TGD people seeking treatments including hormones, and genital, chest, facial and other gender-affirming surgeries require a single written opinion/signature from a health care provider competent to independently assess and diagnose...Further written opinions/signatures may be requested where there is a specific clinical need."[13]

It is essential that providers caring for transgender patients are informed of the historical and generational trauma that transgender patients have been subject to in medical contexts. Although a complete review of the historical trauma of transgender patients in medical contexts is beyond the scope of this article, the fact that transgender patients have been subject to

psychological evaluation before eligibility for medical care is an experience that is more unique to gender-affirming care. In this, there is an assumed and underlying pathology and potential assumptions that transgender people are less entitled to or capable of personal autonomy because they are subject to psychological evaluation and require a licensed mental health providers endorsement before receiving health care.[14]

Providers can mitigate the potential harm of requiring a psychological evaluation before the delivery of surgical services by ensuring that the time spent in the evaluation is of personal benefit for the patient. A partnership directly between the surgical team and the referring mental health provider helps the patient understand the utility of a multidisciplinary approach and benefits the clarity of the treatment plan. Surgical teams can ensure that letters of referral meet the criterion for that surgical clinic as well as pre-authorization needs from the insurance company, though the benefits of referral from a mental health provider exceed administrative processes. Rather, the mental health provider is tasked with defining a psychiatric diagnosis of gender dysphoria and can create a meaningful connection with both the patient and the surgical team by focusing on the psychosocial needs of the patient.

Psychosocial needs of facial surgery patients may include but is not limited to navigating time away from work, school, or care-taking responsibilities (which includes both the financial implications of being away and carefully choosing individuals to take care of tasks while recovering), choosing where to recover such as in a hotel nearby the hospital, at home or at a short-term rental, choosing who can be trusted to care for the patient physically when the patient is recovering (and that may mean multiple people based on their availability or ability to manage the physical demands of caretaking) and discussing with the patient their expectations of the surgery. Mental health providers can also help the patient consider the possibility of revisions or planning for the unexpected, such as a surgical complication that may require more time, money, or patience than originally anticipated.

Given that many TGD patients are subject to undue stress in receiving health care services, it should be anticipated by the surgical team that these patients may have more difficulty advocating for themselves and trusting that the health care provider will be accountable to co-creating a thorough evaluation of the patient's needs and desired outcomes. A mental health provider can help the patient articulate and overcome barriers to advocating for themselves in a surgical context, as well as practice communication with their chosen team to ensure they have awareness and comprehend the need of each medical intervention, have a reasonable ability to speak to their own physical pain and discomfort, and understand the recovery instructions.

In addition, mental health providers should be able to educate the client on signs of post-surgical depression and to plan for unexpected emotions such as sadness, boredom, worry, or frustration which may be common in the immediate days following surgery. Attuned mental health providers also should perform a risk assessment including risk of harm to self, risk of suicidal ideation, risk of abuse of alcohol, and risk of abuse of both prescription and non-prescription drugs. Given that the patient likely has friends or family members who will be present with the patient immediately following surgery, the patient can also discuss with a mental health provider who has been chosen for those tasks and to ensure there is no history of abuse between the patient and those chosen for caretaking, and ensure that the patient is reasonably sure that the chosen caretakers will not use the patient's prescriptions and will protect the dignity of the patient while they are still recovering. In many ways, patients benefit from using mental health services as they undergo major surgical procedures. The challenge for TGD patients is the implication that they are subject to mental health services before proceeding with gender-affirming surgical or medical care, they have the burden to locate the mental health provider largely on their own, and the personal choice to engage in mental health is not offered when the insurer or surgical team requires a mental health referral. Further challenges that TGD patients experience while undergoing surgical care are explored in the following.

BARRIERS IN COVERAGE FOR CARE

The conditions that transgender people are subject to seeking gender-affirming care are also fraught with unnecessary and stressful burdens to the patient. Increasingly, patients seeking gender-affirming care are facing barriers to locating and affording gender affirming care inclusive health insurance.[15] In fact, facial surgeries may be less likely to be a covered service as they are seen as cosmetic by most commercial insurance providers as well as Medicaid providers.[16] Transgender adults are overrepresented as working in settings which do not provide health insurance at all, and many remain underinsured.[17] A contributing factor to the economic stress patients face is that TGD individuals are less likely to have

attended and graduated from college and more likely to live in poverty.[18] The economy available to transgender adults then likely increases the need for patients seeking surgery to raise funds on their own, either to pay in full for surgeries or to cover non-reimbursed expenses. This may include travel to and from the provider's site, time away from work, child or pet care, prescriptions or over-the-counter medications, and the cost of materials for wound care. To increase the trust between providers and patients, a comprehensive estimate of costs for each patient should be provided with resources that can help patients find other means for uncovered services.

FAMILY AND SOCIAL REJECTION

In addition to the financial stress that many transgender patients face, individuals may also face isolation or exclusion from their social or familial communities due to their TGD status. This could exacerbate conditions of depression or anxiety for patients and has been correlated to increased risk of both attempting suicide and misusing drugs and alcohol.[19] Recovery from surgery can be improved when patients are in proximity and support to those persons that they feel most comfortable with. In fact, data suggest that individuals may report diminished physical pain when holding the hand of a loved one,[20] suggesting the importance of TGD patients to have a loved one with them during surgical recovery. For TGD patients who are facing the potential of recovering from surgery without community or family support, they are at an increased risk of presenting to the medical setting in deeper distress. Patients with the means to do so may be able to mitigate their isolation after surgery with hired help such as using a private nurse, though those services are costly and TGD patients also risk bias from those they have called on for help.

Many TGD persons create chosen family systems in which community members, friends, and allies serve as close confidants and may provide a range of support such as financial, emotional, and physical support. TGD patients who present to a surgical context may have a variety of chosen family members that play an important role in that person's life and should be considered an extension of the patient's recovery support team. In some cases, the individuals closest to TGD patients may lack legal status which verifies that they are understood by the patient to be family, nonetheless surgical providers can decrease the stress of TGD patients by addressing supportive chosen family members with the same level of respect as family of origin. Further, TGD people who create chosen family systems but lack support from family of origin remain at an increased risk for developing depression.[21]

INTRUSIVE QUESTIONS ABOUT MEDICAL JOURNEY

An additional level of stress for TGD patients is that transgender individuals face scrutiny for their medical decisions, not just potentially from within the medical and psychological field but also from those in their personal life. Curiosity regarding the medical decisions that transgender patients make is embedded into American culture as media depictions focus on medicalized gender transition and less on the holistic life of TGD people. Transgender patients are not obligated to discuss their personal medical decisions with those outside of their own choosing; however, many TGD individuals report that they are subject to deeply personal and often times offensive lines of questioning from others.[22] This suggests that TGD patients presenting for surgery may have already been subject to a hostile or stressful social environment simply in their pursuit of medical care. Having been predisposed to many levels of interpersonal and systemic stress can create difficulty for the TGD person to arrive at the surgical setting feeling regulated, calm, and with full ability to focus on the medical service.

Finally, TGD patients may hold a variety of additional marginalized identities including racial, ethnic, age, ability, and sexual orientation identities. TGD people who hold additional marginalized identities such as black transgender women are at risk for worse health outcomes due to the impact of racism and misogyny.[23] For patients who are older and are at the beginning of their gender medical transition, they may be at an increased risk of loss of friends or resources due to assumptions about their coming out journeys. Individuals in the lives of older TGD patients may question the need to transition at an older age and may respond with unsupportive or unkind assumptions regarding a person's motivation to transition at a later age.[24] Given the diverse identities of individuals who may present for gender-affirming surgical care, it is important to understand what the specific medical goal is for the patient. For instance, some transgender patients desire to "pass" as their affirmed gender in which it is not evident that they have medically or socially transitioned. For others, passing is not a desired or achievable outcome.[25,26] Hence, plastic surgery providers can decrease the stress of the medical encounter for transgender patients by not assuming the desired outcome of the surgery is to appear cisgender and to carefully consider

and interrupt any risk of bias based on the patient's intersecting identities.

OUTCOMES OF MENTAL HEALTH

Transgender adults may be at risk for adverse health outcomes because of stress related to marginalization and oppression. Forty percent of transgender adults reported attempting suicide at some point in their lifetime, whereas the general adult population in the country reports a lifetime suicide attempt rate at 4.6%.[4] A 2006 study found that suicide attempts in transgender adults was associated with having experiences of recent unemployment, forced sex or rape, verbal and physical victimization related to gender and low self-esteem.[27] In the adult transgender population, both depression and anxiety have been found to surpass the rates of depression and anxiety found in the cisgender population.[28]

Given the relative risk for negative mental health outcomes associated with the discrimination and marginalization of transgender adults, it is important for health care providers to be informed on what can help mitigate negative factors. Gender-affirming medical care has a positive effect on reducing negative mental health problems in transgender patients,[29] though as stated above, the quality of the interaction between the provider and the patient is critical. There is also evidence that gender-affirming facial feminization surgery can improve mental health quality of life for TGD patients.[30] Further, gender-affirming providers should be able to appreciate that mental health symptoms and challenges are not an inherent aspect of being TGD, rather, TGD individuals are subject to intense and multilayered stress, which increases likelihood of developing or worsening mental health disorders.

PROVIDER COMMUNICATION

There are guides to aid surgical providers in reducing both the stress TGD patients experience and thus help to reduce negative mental health outcomes. The following recommendations from the Fenway Health Center[31] can be used to increase effective communication between transgender patients and their medical providers.

- Using a patient's correct name and pronouns
- Maintaining the privacy of patients' gender identities and being careful to only disclose when necessary for care
- Avoiding assumptions about a patient's gender
- Asking only questions pertinent to care (not out of curiosity)

- Admitting inexperience when confronted with an unknown issue or question
- Apologizing for lack of knowledge or making mistakes without offering excuses
- Moving on with the appointment and/or discussion calmly following apology
- Graciously accepting a patient's feedback about unconscious bias, mistakes, or microaggressions

Other guides have suggested the importance of inclusive office procedures which signal support at every step of medical care. For instance, the Transgender Law Center has produced a guide on how to start a transgender clinic[32] and notes that transgender positive posters, literature, and buttons can provide cues that transgender patients are safe at the clinic. Creating a welcoming environment is a key aspect to address the underlying stress that transgender patients often present with to their surgical consultation.

SUMMARY

Addressing the mental health needs of TGD patients who present for gender-affirming facial surgery is a multifaceted task that all members of the clinical and administrative staff can attend to. There is rich opportunity in the surgical setting to offer gender-affirming care that honors the dignity of the patient and acknowledges the multiple layers of systemic and interpersonal stress the patient may have been subject to. Surgical teams benefit the patient as well as the treatment plan when a much broader view of what a health care experience is like from the patient's perspective, which must include the systemic and interpersonal challenges that are more prominent for TGD patients. Finally, medical providers are in a unique position of power to challenge barriers that exist for transgender patients which must begin with acknowledgment that such barriers exist and reduce the quality of care available. Together, all providers that serve TGD patients can choose to eliminate harmful practices which compromise health care outcomes for marginalized patients, and instead offer informed care that is personalized, empowered, and affirming.

CLINICS CARE POINTS

- TGD patients are at risk for negative health outcomes due to increased barriers to care
- Surgical teams should address bias within their institutions
- Surgical teams can improve service delivery by ensuring interactions with patients are equitable
- Collaboration with mental health providers is a key aspect for serving TGD patients

DISCLOSURE

The author has nothing to disclose.

REFERENCES

1. Hidalgo M, Ehrensaft D, Tishelman, et al. The gender affirmative model: what we know and what we aim to learn. Hum Dev 2013;56(5):285–90.
2. Javier C, Crimston Barlow FK, Barlow FK. Surgical satisfaction and quality of life outcomes reported by transgender men and women at least one year post gender-affirming surgery: A systematic literature review. International Journal of Transgender Health 2022;23(3):255–73.
3. Hendricks M, Testa R. A conceptual framework for clinical work with transgender and gender nonconforming clients: An adaptation of the minority stress health model Professional Psychology. Research and Practice 2012;43(5):460–7.
4. James SE, Herman JL, Rankin S, et al. Executive summary of the report of the 2015 U.S. Transgender survey. Washington, DC: National Center for Transgender Equality; 2016.
5. Dhejne C, Lichtenstein P, Boman M, et al. Long-term follow-up of transsexual persons undergoing sex reassignment surgery: Cohort study in Sweden. PLoS One 2011;6:e16885.
6. Clements-Nolle K, Marx R, Mitchell K. Attempted Suicide Among Transgender Persons. J Homosex 2006;51(3):53–69.
7. Patterson CJ, Sepulveda MJ, White J, editors. Understanding the well-being of LGBTQI + populations. Consensus study report. Washington, DC: The National Academies Press; 2020. p. 436.
8. Obedin-Maliver J, Goldsmith ES, Stewart L, et al. Lesbian, gay, bisexual, and transgender-related content in undergraduate medical education. JAMA 2011;306:971–7.
9. Aryanpour Z, Min-Tran D, Ghafoor E, et al. Are we teaching evidence-based and inclusive practices in gender-affirming care? perspectives from plastic surgery in-service examinations. Journal of Graduate Medical Education 2023;15(5):587–91, 1 PMID: 37781442.
10. Von Vogelsang AC, Milton C, Ericsson I, et al. Wouldn't it be easier if you continued to be a guy?' - a qualitative interview study of transsexual persons' experiences of encounters with healthcare professionals. J Clin Nurs 2016;25(23–24):3577–88.

11. Sperber J, Landers S, Lawrence S. Access to healthcare for transgendered persons: Results of a needs assessment in Boston. Int J Transgenderism 2005;8(2–3):75–91.

12. Indyk J, Knuckles K, Hendren V, et al. Ensuring Gender affirming care: Utilizing the electronic health record to improve care of gender-diverse patients in a large pediatric hospital. Pediatrics 2020;146: 304–5.

13. Coleman E, Radix AE, Bouman WP, et al. Standards of Care for the Health of Transgender and Gender Diverse People, Version 8. International Journal of Transgender Health 2022;23(S1):S1–260.

14. Strand N, Jones N. Invisibility of "Gender Dysphoria". AMA Journal of Ethics 2021;23(7): 557–62.

15. Puckett JA, Cleary P, Rossman K, et al. Barriers to gender-affirming care for transgender and gender nonconforming individuals. Sex Res Soc Pol 2018; 15(1):48–59.

16. Gorbea E, Gidumal S, Kozato A, et al. Insurance coverage of facial gender affirmation surgery: a review of medicaid and commercial insurance. Otolaryngol Head Neck Surg 2021;165(6):791–7.

17. Bakko M, Kattari S. Differential Access to Transgender Inclusive Insurance and Healthcare in the United States: Challenges to Health across the Life Course. J Aging Soc Pol 2021;33(1):67–81.

18. Meyer IH, Brown TN, Herman JL, et al. Demographic characteristics and health status of transgender adults in select US regions: behavioral risk factor surveillance system, 2014. Am J Publ Health 2017; 107(4):582–9.

19. Klein A, Golub S. Family rejection as a predictor of suicide attempts and substance misuse among transgender and gender nonconforming adults. LGBT Health 2016;3(3). https://doi.org/10.1089/lgbt.2015.0111.

20. Goldstein P, Weissman-Fogel I, Dumas G, et al. Brain-to-brain coupling during handholding is associated with pain reduction. Proc Natl Acad Sci USA 2018;115(11):201703643.

21. Milton DC, Knutson D. Family of origin, not chosen family, predicts psychological health in a LGBTQ+ sample Psychology of Sexual Orientation and Gender. Diversity 2023;10(2):269–78.

22. Baldwin A, Dodge B, Schick V, et al. Transgender and Genderqueer Individuals' Experiences with Health Care Providers: What's Working, What's Not, and Where Do We Go from Here? J Health Care Poor Underserved 2018;29(4):1300–18. *Project MUSE.*

23. White Hughto JM, Reisner SL, Pachankis JE. Transgender stigma and health: a critical review of stigma determinants, mechanisms, and interventions. Soc Sci Med 2015;147:222–31.

24. Hoy-Ellis CP, Fredriksen-Goldsen KI. Depression among transgender older adults: general and minority stress. Am J Community Psychol 2017;59: 295–305.

25. Anderson AD, Irwin JA, Brown AM, et al. "Your picture looks the same as my picture": an examination of passing in transgender communities. Gend Issues 2020;37:44–60.

26. Clements ZA, Derr BN, Rostosky SS. Male privilege doesn't lift the social status of all men in the same way: Trans masculine individuals' lived experiences of male privilege in the United States. Psychology of Men & Masculinities 2022;23(1):123–32.

27. Clements-Nolle K, Marx R, Katz M. Attempted suicide among transgender persons: The influence of gender-based discrimination and victimization. J Homosex 2006;51:53–69.

28. Budge SL, Adelson JL, Howard KAS. Anxiety and depression in transgender individuals: The roles of transition status, loss, social support, and coping. J Consult Clin Psychol 2013;81(3):545–57.

29. Hughto JMW, Gunn HA, Rood BA, et al. Social and medical gender affirmation experiences are inversely associated with mental health problems in a US non-probability sample of transgender adults. Arch Sex Behav 2020;49(7):2635–47.

30. Ainsworth T, Spiegel J. Quality of life of individuals with and without facial feminization surgery or gender reassignment surgery. Qual Life Res 2010; 19:1019–24.

31. Fenway Health Center National LGBT Health Education Center, Creating a Transgender Health Program at Your Health Center: From Planning to Implementation Sept 2018 https://www.lgbtqiahealtheducation.org/wp-content/uploads/2018/10/Creating-a-Transgender-Health-Program.pdf Accessed October 20, 2023.

32. Transgender Law Center, July 2004 How to start a transgender clinic https://transgenderlawcenter.org/how-to-start-a-transgender-clinic/#:~:text=After%20interviewing%20community%20members%2C%20advocates%2C%20and%20providers%2C%20we,model%20of%20care%20that%20is%20comprehensive%20and%20multi-disciplinary. Accessed October 20, 2023.

Medical Management of Gender Diversity

Corinne S. Heinen, MD[a,b,]*

KEYWORDS

- Gender-affirming • Trauma-informed • Gender dysphoria • Transgender • Nonbinary • Maxillofacial

GLOSSARY

Term	Abbreviation	Definition
Terms used in this article		
Assigned sex at birth	AMAB, AFAB	Assigned male/female at birth as discerned by external examination
Cisgender	CW, CM	Cisgender woman/man; gender identity and sex aligned in most common way seen in society
Gender-affirming		Medical, psychological or surgical care to assist a person have their gender identity and body features/public persona become more congruent
Gender-diverse		All-encompassing term to describe any person whose gender identity or expression does not mesh with social expectations
Gender dysphoria		Psychological distress due to incongruence between gender identity and sex assigned at birth
Nonbinary	NB	Those with transgender identities that do not fit into male and female partitions
Transgender	TGW, TGM	Transgender woman/man; gender identity and sex aligned in and derivative words configuration different from the typical pattern seen in society; implies binary identity
	TF, TM	Transfeminine/masculine, adjectives for identities inclusive of nonbinary persons, sex assigned male/female at birth respectively
	TGD	Transgender and gender diverse
	TGNB	Transgender and gender nonbinary

MEDICAL MANAGEMENT OF GENDER DIVERSITY

Medical care of transgender and gender nonbinary (TGNB) patients is a dynamic field. Similar to gender-affirming surgeries, the evolution of this field is advanced and informed by the needs of gender-diverse patients. Medical and surgical care in concert are needed for many transgender patients to reach sufficient congruence with their gender identity. The aim in this article is to inform oral and maxillofacial surgeons about the concurrent medical care their patients may be receiving

[a] Family Medicine and Internal Medicine, Division of Allergy and Infectious Disease, University of Washington, Seattle, WA, USA; [b] Harborview Medical Center, 325 9th Avenue, Box 359930, Seattle, WA 98104, USA
* Harborview Medical Center, 325 9th Avenue, Box 359930, Seattle, WA 98104.
E-mail address: cheinen@uw.edu

Oral Maxillofacial Surg Clin N Am 36 (2024) 151–159
https://doi.org/10.1016/j.coms.2023.12.005
1042-3699/24/© 2023 Elsevier Inc. All rights reserved.

oralmaxsurgery.theclinics.com

and to identify ways that gender-affirming medical and surgical care may interrelate.

BACKGROUND

Sex, gender identity, and gender expression are separate components of the human experience; all occur on a spectrum. Gender identity encompasses a core sense of self that involves perspectives, emotions, societal role, and social interaction. For many, this sense of self does not fit into the circumscribed, dichotomous spheres of masculine and feminine identities but rather is on a continuum. People who experience their identity in an intermediate space may use self-descriptors of having gender nonbinary or genderqueer identities. Gender expression describes how a person presents to the world via dress, hairstyle, manner, voice, and other outward representation.

Transgender and gender-diverse (TGD; is inclusive of a broader set of identities than TGNB) people comprise an enduring subpopulation of humankind, with documentation of their existence dating back thousands of years. Some civilizations have had specific societal roles at the community or familial level for gender-diverse members. Current estimates from the US Census Bureau's Household Pulse Survey show that the approximately 0.6% of the adult population of the United States identify as transgender.[1]

There is no current explanation for the differing associations between gender identity and sex. Reproductive organs form during the first trimester of pregnancy, whereas the brain develops throughout the prenatal period and beyond. Greater insight into influences over these varied time frames of maturation may eventually shed light on why people are transgender, nonbinary, or cisgender. Regardless, our task is to assist with the health and well-being of the patients under our care.

CONTEXT FOR THE LIVES OF TRANSGENDER AND GENDER NONBINARY PEOPLE
Realization of Transgender Identity

Insight into the experiences of gender-diverse people enhances our ability to provide the best care. Many are aware of the discordance between their gender identity and sex (as compared to the alignment seen in cisgender individuals) early in life. Children usually identify as a girl or a boy by age 3. For some, the dissonance between gender identity and sex assigned at birth rises to the level of awareness at the outset of puberty when unwelcome bodily changes occur.[2] Given the many tasks of development and the influences of environmental factors, self-awareness of being gender

diverse may not occur until adulthood. Those who are transgender, nonbinary, or otherwise gender diverse may delay revealing their identity to others for years or even decades to avoid social repercussions.

By the time adults present for gender-affirming care, their decision has often been long-considered. Gender identity can represent an evolving understanding, however, so there can be elements of ongoing discernment. This may occur when patients start gender-affirming medications, as the change in their internal milieu can create plasticity in their self-understanding, as in any puberty.

Social and Physical Transition

There is no singular path for a person to move through gender transition. Most TGNB individuals will go through social transition as a first step, which includes disclosure of their identity to others; requesting to be addressed by applicable pronouns; and often by changing their name. Some will change their legal name and documents, but not all have the resources to do so.

Physical transition is another common step, which involves changing one's gender expression, as mentioned earlier. It may include hair removal by electrolysis or laser. Transmasculine individuals (masculine identity, inclusive of nonbinary persons, sex assigned female at birth [AFAB]; hereafter TM) may wear chest binders to minimize contours of chest tissue. To be clear, an individual does not need to follow a specific template for transition or present in a given way to prove that they are TGNB. A patient's gender expression sometimes may not fit with a provider's expectations; recognize that our notions may spring from societal norms that may not be relevant to the person before us.

MEDICAL TRANSITION
Diagnosis and Principles of Management

To qualify for medical or surgical treatment, a patient must meet the criteria for the diagnosis of gender dysphoria. The Diagnostic and Statistical Manual of Mental Disorders, Fifth Edition (DSM-V) criteria are concise, specific and straightforward to interpret (**Table 1**).[3] The standard of care is that a medical provider makes the diagnosis of gender dysphoria in adults according to DSM-V criteria; except in complex cases, a separate mental health evaluation is not indicated. If the criteria are met and have been in place for longer than 6 months, treatment is offered (termed the informed consent model).[4–6] Counseling on risks and benefits, as well as treating

Table 1
Diagnostic and Statistical Manual of Mental Disorders, Fifth Edition criteria for gender dysphoria in adults

Marked incongruence between gender identity and sex assigned at birth, which has been present for 3 mo & has 2 more of the following:	• Marked incongruence between experienced/expressed gender and primary/secondary sex characteristics • Strong desire to get rid of primary/secondary sex characteristics due to incongruence with experienced/expressed gender • Stronger desire for primary/secondary sex characteristics of the other gender • Strong desire to be of other gender • Strong desire to be treated as the other gender • Strong conviction that one has the typical feelings and reactions of the other gender
And the condition is associated with clinically significant distress or impairment in social, occupational, or other important areas of functioning	

comorbidities prior to or concurrently with the beginning of gender-affirming medications, is required.[5]

To provide the most effective care, both gender-affirming surgical and medical providers require insight into a patient's identity. Whether cisgender or transgender, all people value certain attributes as most important to their presentation to the world. Eliciting a patient's particular priorities is key to guiding treatment decisions.[4]

Gender-affirming medical care focuses on alleviating gender dysphoria by de-emphasizing body features that indicate the patient's sex assigned at birth and promoting acquisition of secondary sexual characteristics concordant with their gender identity. Sometimes both can be achieved by a single medication, such as the use of spironolactone to lessen body hair while simultaneously adding to breast development. Estradiol and testosterone induce secondary sexual characteristics effectively but have only limited ability to lessen established traits. For instance, the anatomy of laryngeal cords does not change in response to estradiol, nor does breast tissue significantly atrophy for those on testosterone.[7]

The pluripotential nature of the embryo as it relates to sex development allows either estradiol or testosterone to feed back to the hypothalamic-pituitary-gonadal axis. Intake of estradiol downregulates endogenous production of testosterone and vice versa. Estradiol and testosterone induce the development of secondary sexual characteristics that are consonant with patient goals while diminishing the release of intrinsic sex hormones (**Fig. 1**).

Initiation of Gender Affirming Medications

In transfeminine (feminine identity, inclusive of nonbinary persons, sex assigned male at birth;

hereafter TF) individuals, estradiol will induce breast development and soften the skin. In TM individuals, development of a lower voice, increased lean body mass, more facial and body hair, and attenuation or cessation of menses are

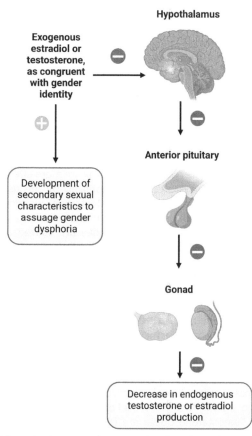

Fig. 1. Downregulation of the hypothalamic-pituitary-gonadal axis by exogenous sex hormones in the medical management of gender dysphoria. (Created with BioRender.com.)

characteristic changes. Some body attributes are on a spectrum, such as fat distribution tending toward a bimodal pattern. Early in treatment, there may be diminishment/increase of libido in TF/TM patients; however, these differences revert toward the mean over time.[8]

It is extremely helpful to patients to counsel them about the anticipated time course of evolution of secondary sexual characteristics. Transgender women (identifies as a woman in a binary way, assigned male at birth, hereafter TGW) have early changes to skin and muscle mass, but breast development can take 2 to 3 years. Transgender men (converse, hereafter TGM) are generally pleased that their voices will lower within 6 to 12 months; having the context that complete clitoral enlargement may take 2 years is reassuring in the meantime. Please refer the Endocrine Society Guidelines for details.[6]

Before starting gender-affirming hormonal treatment (GAHT), information is given about irreversible features that persist off medications, such as a lowered voice or the presence of breast tissue. Fertility may be permanently affected; this cannot be ascertained in advance. If a patient wishes to preserve future fertility, storing gametes is recommended.

Differing formulations of sex hormones are available. Safety and efficacy are primary concerns in the discussion between the patient and the clinician. Logistical concerns such as cost, formulary, ease of titration, acceptability of using needles, or contact dermatitis affect choice of formulation. For some, it is easier to remember to use a topical application daily, while for others weekly injections are more facile. Some formulations are more effective for achieving changes prioritized by the patient, such as injectable testosterone working better than gel to attain amenorrhea.[9]

Both testosterone and estradiol are started at approximately one-quarter of the maximum dose and increased incrementally, seldom more quickly than every 3 months. Longer intervals between titration steps are beneficial to assess changes that require more time to evolve.[6] Slower increases may be used if there is concern for potential side effects, for example, migraines in TF patients with a family history of the same. Nonbinary patients may wish to advance the dose slowly to assess their response at each level. Using the lowest effective dose is safest, though this must be weighed against the urgency to achieve relief of gender dysphoria.

Testosterone doses are in the same range as would be used for replacement therapy in hypogonadal cisgender men (CM). For many TM patients, the optimal dose is lower than the possible maximum. However, the estradiol dosing needed to suppress testosterone production is 2 to 4 times higher than the replacement dose for premenopausal cisgender women (CW), and the use of near-maximal doses is often required. Lower doses suffice after orchiectomy.[10]

Gender-Affirming Hormone Dosing

With these principles in mind, the following table lists the doses of sex hormones that are most commonly used. Only medication formulations available in the United States are listed. The goal of treatment is to relieve dysphoria not to treat to a specific hormonal level. Hormone levels help ensure a patient is staying within safe ranges. Common estradiol preparations are listed (**Table 2**).

Testosterone dosing falls within the following parameters. There are some known effects on the efficacy of different formulations. Injectable testosterone is more effective at suppressing menses. Subcutaneous and topical testosterone are less like to cause erythrocytosis (**Table 3**).[7,11] Testosterone formulations that are less frequently used are not listed in the chart: nasal gel and oral testosterone undecanoate.

Adjunctive Gender-Affirming Medications

The combination of sex hormones and adjunctive medications comprise the full set of options for gender-affirming medical therapy (GAMT). Adjunctive medications are used mostly for feminization. Spironolactone has been used as an androgen blocker and adds some assistance with breast development. The effects of progesterone are still not well characterized, so it is not recommended by guidelines, but some individuals feel that it assists with aspects of breast development. Micronized progesterone is safest as progestins increase thrombogenic risk. Gonadotropin hormone-releasing hormone analogues effectively prevent the production of endogenous hormones, but their use is limited by expense and the need for injections or implants for administration. Dutasteride and finasteride are used by both TF/TM individuals for preservation of scalp hair.

Neither the hormones nor adjunctive medications prescribed for gender-affirming care should affect bleeding or infection risk. Proactively letting patients know that antibiotics or other prescriptions will not interfere with the effects of GAMT will ensure greater adherence.

Side Effects of Gender-Affirming Medical Treatment

Cancer risk
There is no increased risk of common cancers known to result from testosterone use. Several

Table 2
Options for feminizing hormone therapy

	Feminizing Hormone Therapy		
Medication	Formulations	Dosing	Comments
Estradiol 17-beta estradiol	Transdermal	0.1–0.4 mg/day	Transdermal use has lowest VTE risk. More costly At times contact dermatitis or will not adhere
Estradiol 17-beta estradiol	Oral	Starting: 1 mg Maximum: 6–8 mg If dosing 2 mg take daily; split to bid if > 2 mg	Higher VTE risk than transdermal Conjugated estrogens and ethinyl estradiol should not be used due to VTE risk
Estradiol valerate Estradiol cypionate }Not equipotent		IM 5–20 mg weekly IM 1.25–5 mg	Some feel this is more efficacious than other formulations. Frequent supply chain difficulties

Abbreviations: IM, intramuscular; VTE, venous thromboembolism.

studies have shown both TGW and TGM have an increased risk of breast cancer intermediate between CW and CM, though some showed similar rates between TGM and CW. There is no apparent increase in ovarian, uterine, or cervical cancer in TGM due to testosterone use compared to CW.[12] A meta-analysis of TF individuals on gender-affirming hormone therapy noted that all published cohort studies have described a lower incidence of prostate cancer in them compared to CM.[13] There are rare benign brain tumors that can occur with greater frequency on GAHT: prolactinoma in TGW and somatotrophinoma in TGM.[14]

Metabolic conditions
Cross-sectional studies show bone health is preserved in transgender adults undergoing GAHT, although adherence to hormone replacement is critical in those who have had gonadectomy. TGM have normal bone density over the life span; TGW have higher rates of osteoporosis but also have lower relative bone mineral density before starting GAHT.[15]

When a cohort of TM were followed longitudinally, an increase in lean mass was observed with testosterone therapy with a reduction in body fat.[16] The converse has been seen in TF.[17] Insulin resistance

Table 3
Options for masculinizing hormone therapy

	Masculinizing Hormone Therapy		
Medication	Formulations	Dosing	Comments
Testosterone	Gel (1% or 1.62%)	20–100 mg daily	Can transfer to others. More gradual effects. Does not suppress menses as well
	Intramuscular/ Subcutaneous (testosterone enanthate or cypionate; equipotent)	25–100 mg weekly/up to 200 biweekly	Subcutaneous must be dosed weekly, Intramuscular can stretch to 10–14 d
	Patch (testosterone)	2–6 mg qd (1–3 patches)	Contact dermatitis
	Pellets	Implanted every 3 mo	Limited dosing flexibility Pellets do not need to be removed
	Testosterone undecanoate (also oral form but recommended only for Klinefelter's)	Intramuscular at clinic q 10 wk	Possible lung effects

was unchanged in TGM and increased in TGW. Prospective studies have shown low-density lipoprotein (LDL) and triglycerides increased and high-density lipoprotein HDL decreased in TGM after starting testosterone. TGW had decreased LDL. Those on oral estradiol had increased fasting insulin levels and decreased HDL while those on transdermal estradiol did not have significant changes.[17,18]

Cardiovascular disease and venous thromboembolism

A retrospective study reviewing 43 years of records discerned TGW had more strokes and venous thromboembolism (VTE) compared to CW, CM, and TGM. This risk can be greatly influenced by dose and formulation of medication. In feminizing care, oral 17 beta-estradiol likely represents a higher risk of VTE relative to patches.[19] Ethinyl estradiol and conjugated estrogens are not used for GAHT; they are more thrombogenic than 17 beta-estradiol. The same study showed a significantly higher occurrence of myocardial infarction in TGW and TGM undergoing testosterone treatment compared to CW, but CM had the most myocardial infarctions relative to all groups.[20]

Psychological outcomes

A review of 19 prospective studies on the psychological effects of GAHT showed improvements in depression and psychological distress in both TF and TM people. Effects on anxiety varied across sources. Cross-sectional investigations evaluated in the same review indicated decreased social anxiety in TM on GAHT.[21]

THE CONTINUUM BETWEEN MEDICAL AND SURGICAL CARE
Effects of Medical Management on Facial Appearance

Medical management has finite benefits for facial changes in TGD people seeking better congruence between their physical traits and gender identity. Testosterone promotes facial hair, though can it take 5 years for maximal effect.[7] Facial muscle may increase in TGM.[22] Unfortunately, estradiol and spironolactone have limited ability to diminish facial hair.

The shape of the face is only modestly altered by gender-affirming hormone therapy. A study using 3-dimensional modeling demonstrated that changes in fat redistribution can be seen by 3 months after start and continued to evolve over the 12 months of the study. On estradiol, there is more prominence of the cheeks and less so of the jaw; the converse is seen with testosterone. It is not known when these changes plateau.[23] Of note, pretreatment with hormonal therapy is not required prior to gender-affirming facial surgeries as per the World Professional Association for Transgender Health guidelines but hormonally induced facial changes can impact the ultimate surgical decision-making for those seeking gender-affirming facial surgery.[5]

Anesthesia

Oral and maxillofacial surgeons have the additional skill of providing anesthesia as well as performing surgery. Here are some factors that may influence readiness for surgery and perioperative course of gender-diverse patients.

- There are no interactions between gender-affirming medications and anesthesia or antibiotics that would be used in the setting of oral and maxillofacial surgery procedures.[24] To promote adherence, it is important to assure patients that prescribed medications for aftercare will not interfere with GAHT.
- Chest binders are elastic garments that compress tissue against the chest wall to minimize tissue prominence and lessen gender dysphoria. Binders could increase resistance to inhalation for patients undergoing conscious sedation. Prior to requesting removal, if necessary, explain the medical concerns and ensure the patient can don their binder quickly postoperatively to promote both medical and psychological safety.[24,25]
- People who were AFAB have a smaller airway diameter. Testosterone enables obstructive sleep apnea both anatomically and physiologically even in young individuals, which could increase airway resistance in those receiving general anesthesia.

Laboratory Values

Creatinine, alkaline phosphatase, hemoglobin, and hematocrit do vary based on sex hormone use. Interpret the normal range based on the laboratory range consistent with the sex hormone being utilized.[11]

APPROACH TO PATIENTS WHO ARE GENDER DIVERSE
Current Transgender and Gender-Diverse Experiences in the Dental Setting

Dental procedures can be difficult for many people. This apprehension is elevated in people who fear or have experienced inattentive or negative treatment previously in health care settings, which unfortunately has been a common experience for TGNB people.

A cross-sectional survey showed a slightly higher score on the Dental Fear Survey in TGW and TGM compared to historical cisgender comparators. Gender-nonconforming patients had much higher scores. Patients with unconventional gender expression may experience awkward interactions with clinicians more frequently. The gender-nonconforming group had significantly higher scores on the avoidance of care subscale.[26]

Another study queried TGD patients about their priorities and experiences in dental settings. One-third of the participants reported misgendering (having been addressed by an incorrect name or pronoun) although being correctly addressed was listed as a priority. More than one-half felt their usual source of oral health care was not equipped to provide gender-appropriate care. In this study, 48% of the participants reported avoiding the dentist at least occasionally because of unease about how they would be treated.[27]

Trauma-Informed Care in the Oral and Maxillofacial Surgery Setting

The precepts of trauma-informed care (TIC) were created to guide clinicians to intentionally create a sense of safety for patients. This approach enhances the care for anyone with a history of trauma but also applies to those who feel vulnerable to prejudicial treatment in care settings given larger societal patterns. Incorporating these tools into daily practice is ideal for all patients.

An approach to TIC in the dental setting is described in the work by Raja and colleagues.[28] Suggested practical actions included proactively asking for ways to help make a person more comfortable, using the tell-show-do approach, and giving patients the option of having a signal to pause during a procedure. These are excellent, universal examples of ways to avoid invoking or creating a traumatic experience.

Following are primary tenets of TIC, followed by specific applications for care of gender-diverse individuals.

- *Be life and identity affirming.*
  - Use current name and pronouns in all settings and in the record. Have these easily visible in the chart.
  - If the legal name differs from the current name, never state the legal name (aka, dead name) out loud; allow visual verification instead.
  - Apologize sincerely but concisely if you misstate a name or pronoun. Thank the person if they inform you of your error.
  - Query current name, pronouns, gender identity, and sex assigned at birth on intake forms, with blank areas for pronouns and gender identity. Allow for entry of this information in your patient portal.

- Avoid gendered titles like Mr or Ms unless a specific patient prefers to be addressed in this way.
- *Elicit the patient's needs, rather than assuming them.* TGNB patients may have differing perspectives than expected on their goal when seeking gender-affirming surgeries. A TM, nonbinary patient may or may not desire a typically male jawline.
- *Offer the patient agency and choice*
  - Be transparent about options for their care.
  - If a patient needs to pause a procedure, honor their request.
  - Ensure the patient gives the final word on decisions.
- *Make the environment feel as safe as possible*
  - Pronoun pins or badge buddies show you are familiar with TGNB experiences.
  - Mark single-use bathrooms as gender neutral. Multi-stall bathroom signs should indicate that anyone may use the bathroom concordant with their gender identity.
  - Welcome the presence of accompanying support people.
- Recall that patients who have experienced trauma in the past may act reactive or withdrawn. Give grace and space if this occurs, as they are likely responding to anxiety or invoked memories.[22,29,30]

SUMMARY

Awareness exists that altered appearance after injury or cancer can itself be disabling, affecting a person's ability to function in the society. Similarly, incongruence between stated gender and residual traits from sex assigned at birth can create impediments in the interpersonal interactions of TGD people. The techniques outlined in the remainder of this volume outline the transformative tools available to oral and maxillofacial surgeons to assist transgender and gender-diverse patients to move forward with their lives.

CLINICS CARE POINTS

- Being aware of the medical background and life experiences of gender-diverse patients can make oral and maxillofacial care more facile for the surgeon and more therapeutic for the patient.
- The most common medications used in medical management of gender dysphoria include testosterone for TM patients and estradiol, finasteride, and spironolactone in TF individuals.

None should affect bleeding or infection risk, nor interact with anesthetic agents.

- Surgical care for treatment of gender dysphoria related to facial features is key as medical treatment has limited effects.
- Attention to ensuring a sense of safety for patients and other trauma-informed approaches enhance communication and quality of care.

ACKNOWLEDGMENTS

Acknowledgments to Remigio A. Roque, MD, and Geoffrey M. Greenlee, DDS, MSD, MPH.

DISCLOSURE

The author has nothing to disclose.

REFERENCES

1. Anderson L, File T, Marshall J, et al. New household pulse survey data reveals differences between LGBT and non-LGBT respondents during COVID-19 pandemic. 2021. Available at: https://www.census.gov/library/stories/2021/11/census-bureau-survey-explores-sexual-orientation-and-gender-identity.html. Accessed July 15, 2023.
2. Misakian A, Mehringer J. Transgender and gender diverse youth. In: Tenney-Soeiro R, Devon E, editors. Netter's pediatrics. 2nd edition. Philadelphia: Elsevier; 2023. p. 97–9.
3. American Psychiatric Association. Diagnostic and statistical manual of mental disorders. 5th edition. Arlington, VA: American Psychiatric Publishing; 2013.
4. Deutsch M. Use of the informed consent model in the provision of cross-sex hormone therapy: A survey of the practices of selected clinics. Int J Transgenderism 2011;13:140–6.
5. Coleman E, Radix A, Bouman WP, et al. (2022) Standards of care for the health of transgender and gender diverse people, version 8. International Journal of Transgender Health 2022;23:S31–40.
6. Cavanaugh T, Hopwood R, Lambert C. Informed consent in the medical care of transgender and gender-nonconforming patients. AMA J Ethics 2016;18(11):1147–55.
7. Wylie C, Cohen-Kettenis PT, Gooren L, et al. Endocrine treatment of gender-dysphoric/gender-incongruent persons: an Endocrine Society clinical practice guideline. J Clin Endocrinol Metabol 2017;102(11):3869–903.
8. Defreyne J, Elaut E, Kreukels B, et al. Sexual desire changes in transgender individuals upon initiation of hormone treatment. J Sex Med 2020;17(4):812–25.
9. Defreyne J, Vanwonterghema Y, Collet Y, et al. Vaginal bleeding and spotting in transgender men after initiation of testosterone therapy: a prospective cohort study (ENIGI). Int J Transgend Health 2020 February 12;21(2):163–75.
10. Gooren L, Giltay E, Bunck M. Long-term treatment of transsexuals with cross-sex hormones: extensive personal experience. J Clin Endocrinol Metab 2008;93(1):19–25.
11. Deutsch, M. Guidelines for the primary and gender-affirming care of transgender and gender nonbinary people. 2016. Available at https://transcare.ucsf.edu/guidelines. Accessed July 15, 2023.
12. Leone A, Trapani D, Schabath M, et al. Cancer in transgender and gender-diverse persons: a review. JAMA Oncol 2023;9(4):556–63.
13. Tanaka M, Sahota K, Burn J, et al. Prostate cancer in transgender women: what does a urologist need to know? BJU Int 2022;129:113–22.
14. Nota N, Wiepjes C, de Blok C, et al. The occurrence of benign brain tumours in transgender individuals during cross-sex hormone treatment. Brain 2018;141:2047–54.
15. Lewiecki EM, Anderson PA, Bilezikian JP, et al. Proceedings of the 2021 Santa Fe bone symposium: advances in the management of osteoporosis and metabolic bone diseases. J Clin Densitom 2022;25:3–19.
16. Pirtea P, Ayoubi JM, Desmedt S, et al. Ovarian, breast, and metabolic changes induced by androgen treatment in transgender men. Fertil Steril 2021;116(4):536–42.
17. Klaver M, Dekker M, de Mutsert R, et al. Cross-sex hormone therapy in transgender persons affects total body weight, body fat and lean body mass: a meta-analysis. Andrologia 2017;49(5):e12660.
18. Wiesckx K, Van Caenegem E, Schreiner T, et al. Cross-sex hormone therapy in trans persons is safe and effective at short-time follow-up. J Sex Med 2014;11:1999–2011.
19. Rovinski D, Ramos R, Fighera T, et al. Risk of venous thromboembolism events in postmenopausal women using oral versus non-oral hormone therapy: a systematic review and meta-analysis. Thromb Res 2018;168:83–95.
20. Nota N, Wiepjes C, de Blok C, et al. Occurrence of acute cardiovascular events in transgender individuals receiving hormone therapy. Circulation 2019;139:1461–2.
21. Doyle D, Lewis, Barreto M. A systematic review of psychosocial functioning changes after gender-affirming hormone therapy among transgender people. Nat Human Behav 2023.
22. Esmonde N, Najafian A, Penkin A, et al. The role of facial gender confirmation surgery in the treatment of gender dysphoria. J Craniofac Surg 2019;30:1387–92.
23. Tebbens M, Nota N, Liberton N, et al. Treatment induces facial feminization in transwomen and masculinization in transmen: quantification by 3D scanning

and patient-reported outcome measures. J Sex Med 2019;16:746e754.

24. Tollinche L, Walters C, Radix A, et al. The perioperative care of the transgender patient 2018;127(2):359–66.

25. Roque R. Transgender pediatric surgical patients-important perioperative considerations. Pediatric Anesthesia 2020;00:1–9.

26. Heima M, Heaton L, Ng H, et al. Dental fear among transgender individuals - a cross-sectional survey 2017;37(5):212–22.

27. Raisin J, Keels M, Roberts M, et al. Barriers to oral health care for transgender and gender nonbinary populations. JADA 2023;154(5):384–92.

28. Raja S, Hoersch M, Rajagopalan C, et al. Treating patients with traumatic life experiences: providing trauma-informed care. J Am Dent Assoc 2014; 145(3):238–45.

29. Tamrat J. "Trans-forming" dental practice norms: Exploring transgender identity and oral health implications. Can J Dent Hyg 2022;56(3):131–9.

30. Substance Abuse and Mental Health Services Administration. SAMHSA's Concept of trauma and guidance for a trauma-informed approach. HHS publication No. (SMA) 14-4884. Rockville, MD: Substance Abuse and Mental Health Services Administration; 2014.

Surgical Standards of Care and Insurance Authorization of Gender-Affirming Facial Surgery

Danielle Eble, MD[a],*, Emily Hem[b]

KEYWORDS

- Gender affirming surgery • Facial feminization • Facial masculinization • Insurance authorization

KEY POINTS

- Recent legislation has expanded insurance coverage of gender-affirming surgeries, yet transgender and gender-diverse patients still face multifactorial barriers to care.
- Facial gender-affirming surgeries are considered uniquely "cosmetic" procedures by many insurers and are therefore less likely to be covered than other types of gender-affirming surgeries.
- Health care professionals must be well-versed in the World Professional Association for Transgender Health Standards of Care to best deliver high-quality care to transgender and gender-diverse patients.
- The Standards of Care inform insurance policies, yet key differences exist between these guidelines and certain insurance requirements.
- Insurance authorization for facial gender-affirming surgery is a complex, highly variable process that requires meticulous surgeon documentation, comprehensive letters of support attesting to medical and mental health clearance, and a highly experienced administrative support team to circumnavigate denials.

INTRODUCTION

There has been striking growth in the transgender and gender-diverse (TGD) population in recent years. Between 2017 and 2020, at least 1.3 million adults and 300,000 youth have identified as transgender in the United States.[1] Accordingly, unprecedented demand for medically necessary gender-affirming interventions has impacted the current landscape of health care legislation, research, and practice standards. Yet many TGD patients still face complex, multifactorial barriers to care. Insurance coverage for gender-affirming surgery (GAS) is one such obstacle, as payer denials and coverage gaps can delay or prohibit patients from accessing these procedures. Providers must therefore understand the nuances of insurance policy and procedure to optimize patient safety and access to GAS.

Historically, TGD patients were largely required to pay out of pocket for GAS, despite being disproportionately low-income and unemployed compared to the general population.[2] However, the passage of the Affordable Care Act (ACA) in 2010 extended universal health care to previously uninsured populations, including TGD patients seeking GAS. Subsequent provisions to the ACA specifically prohibited insurance and health care discrimination against TGD patients, further expanding third-party

[a] Division of Plastic Surgery, Department of Surgery, University of Washington, 325 9th Avenue, Mailstop 359796, Seattle, WA 98104, USA; [b] Division of Plastic Surgery, Department of Surgery, University of Washington, 325 9th Avenue, Mailstop 359835, Seattle, WA 98104, USA
* Corresponding author.
E-mail address: deble@uw.edu

Oral Maxillofacial Surg Clin N Am 36 (2024) 161–169
https://doi.org/10.1016/j.coms.2023.12.004
1042-3699/24/Published by Elsevier Inc.

coverage of GAS. This legislation contributed to a 109% and 392% increase in feminizing and masculinizing procedures from 2015 to 2018, respectively.[3]

It is important to note that the ACA nondiscrimination clause has been politically schismatic on local and national levels. This has resulted in highly variable third-payer coverage of GAS, particularly for Medicaid recipients. As of 2020, 18 states offered some level of gender-affirming coverage for Medicaid patients, whereas 13 states explicitly denied coverage for these services.[4] Similarly, Medicaid recipients are more likely to be denied GAS or have no in-network providers than patients who are privately insured, illustrating an additional point of inequity for low-income or unemployed TGD patients.[5]

The legislative divide between GAS advocates and dissenters has widened in recent years. While some states have expanded protections for TGD persons, others have actively denounced and revoked the rights of this population. In 2022 alone, 26 anti-trans bills were signed into law in 13 states, including Alabama's passage of the first bill imposing criminal penalties on health care professionals who provide gender-affirming care.[6] This legislation imposes unique challenges on TGD patients who must cross state lines to pursue care in nonpunitive areas, which may further affect coverage status.

Facial gender affirming surgery (FGAS) is a critical component of TGD health care that is strongly associated with psychosocial and quality of life benefits due to improvements in both self-perception and public perception.[7–9] Despite the growing body of literature supporting the medical necessity of FGAS, most insurers uniquely categorize these procedures as cosmetic. Consequentially, FGAS is less likely to be acknowledged or reimbursed compared to body-affirming procedures. A 2020 policy review found that FGAS was mentioned in only 17% of state Medicaid policies with GAS coverage. Similarly, 51% of commercial insurers with a published policy on FGAS identified these procedures as cosmetic. This represents a stark contrast to genital-affirming surgery, which was categorized as medically necessary by 100% of commercial insurance policies with GAS coverage.[4] Despite demonstrable disparities in FGAS coverage, nearly two-thirds of facial feminization surgery (FFS) cases between 2015 and 2017 were reimbursed through Medicaid or private insurers and nearly half of all FFS patients were below the 50th percentile for income.[10] Existing comprehensive policies, although not in the majority, unquestionably improve equity and access to FGAS.

DISCUSSION
The Standards of Care for Gender-Affirming Surgery

The World Professional Association for Transgender Health (WPATH) is an international organization comprised of over 3000 multidisciplinary medicolegal professionals dedicated to transgender health care, research, policy, and advocacy. In their founding year of 1979, WPATH developed the first evidence-based clinical guidelines promoting uniform, high-quality health care for TGD patients, known as the Standards of Care (SOC). Seven additional versions of the SOC have since been published, reflecting evolving scientific literature and medical practices—most recently in September 2022 with the SOC-8.[11,12]

The SOC-8 outlines practice standards for medical providers who recommend or perform GAS, including patient candidacy, that ultimately inform procedural coverage by insurers.[13] Failure to meet these standards threatens patient safety and may result in unnecessary delays in care. Health care professionals must therefore be well-versed in the SOC-8 to ensure compatible preoperative work-up and documentation.

First and foremost, multidisciplinary health professionals must be trained to care for TGD individuals specifically. The SOC-8 mandates that providers be licensed by their respective statutory body, at least holding a master's degree or equivalent clinical training. Professionals involved with TGD care should have experience assessing gender dysphoria, incongruence, diversity, and co-existing mental health or psychosocial concerns. Providers are similarly expected to have competency using the World Health Organization's International Classification of Diseases (ICD) for diagnosis and with assessing a patient's capacity to consent for treatment. Finally, the SOC-8 encourages health professionals to work with a multidisciplinary team when assessing patients for gender-affirming procedures and to pursue continuing education on related topics.[12]

Similarly, the SOC-8 outlines a comprehensive set of criteria that patients must meet prior to undergoing GAS, including facial feminization and masculinization. These medicolegal requirements involve documentation of sustained gender incongruence, thorough capacity assessments, and multidisciplinary medical and psychiatric clearance.[12] The process is lengthy, rigorous, and intentional to promote patient safety and satisfaction and minimize decisional regret.[14–17]

Sustained, well-documented gender incongruence is perhaps the most strongly emphasized

SOC-8 requirement amongst patients considering any gender-affirming medical or surgical intervention. Gender incongruence is defined as an incompatibility between an individual's psychological sense of gender and their assigned sex at birth.[12] Gender incongruence may contribute to mental or physical distress, known as gender dysphoria, but it is important to differentiate between these two conditions.[18] The ICD 11th edition formally recognizes "gender incongruence of adolescence and adulthood" as a disorder of sexual health, rather than mental ill-health. This terminology replaces obsolete diagnoses from the 10th edition, such as "transsexualism," "transvestism," and "gender identity disorder," thereby destigmatizing the TGD population.[19]

Gender incongruence is commonly diagnosed by an experienced primary care or mental health provider prior to surgical consultation. Although patients must demonstrate sustained gender incongruence, there is no specified duration of time that supports a clinical diagnosis. Health professionals are therefore encouraged to perform a holistic assessment of the patient's gender identity and the nature and persistence of their incongruence. Supportive documents include government-issued identification and medical records reflective of one's preferred gender identity. Public changes in gender expression, name, or pronouns can also be considered. It is important to note that many patients experience gender incongruence privately and therefore lack objective evidence of an alternate gender identity. Thus, in situations where no documentation is available or a sudden change in gender-identity is suspected, longitudinal observation is recommended to confirm stability prior to initiating gender-affirming treatments.[12]

As with all surgeries, preprocedural evaluation for GAS should also include a holistic assessment of the patient's medical, psychiatric, and social comorbidities to inform discussion of surgical risk and benefit. In general, access to gender-affirming care should not be delayed due to the overwhelming benefit of these interventions on patients' mental and physical health. Exceptions include patients who are unable to engage in the process of transition, provide informed consent, and safely manage postsurgical care, as well as those who have unacceptable operative risk due to pre-existing conditions.[12]

Capacity to consent is of paramount importance when considering GAS, as these procedures may irreversibly affect one's appearance, fertility, and sexual function. Patients must have the cognitive capacity to understand and retain potential positive and negative outcomes of the surgery and use this information to synthesize an informed decision about whether or not to proceed. Patients must also be at the age of majority in their country to undergo most types of GAS, including FGAS.[12]

Surgeon Consultation and Documentation for Facial Gender-Affirming Surgeries

Surgeons must systematically assess and document patients' candidacy for FGAS to meet insurance requirements. While the WPATH SOC guides insurance policies, there are key differences for surgeons to be aware of when submitting for procedural authorization and coverage. For example, the SOC-8 focuses heavily on gender incongruence as the primary measure of patient readiness for gender-affirming interventions.[12] While gender incongruence is a component of insurance criteria, a diagnosis of persistent, well-documented gender dysphoria—or distress related to one's gender incongruence—is the crux of most policies. Similarly, hormone therapy is not a specific requirement for FGAS based on the SOC-8, but many insurers consider gender-affirming pharmacotherapies to be an objective measure of sustained gender incongruence.[12]

Surgeon documentation should therefore focus heavily on the patient's diagnosis of gender dysphoria and the medical necessity of FGAS. Providers are recommended to document patients' assigned sex at birth, gender identity, pronouns, and duration living in their current gender identity full-time. A diagnosis of gender dysphoria should be explicitly noted. This diagnosis is made by the patient's longitudinal medical or mental health professional prior to surgical consultation. However, surgeons should substantiate the patient's diagnosis of gender dysphoria by documenting prior gender-affirming interventions—including duration and effects of hormone therapy and self-identified facial and vocal characteristics that trigger dysphoria. Surgeons may further validate the medical necessity of FGAS by capturing how the patient's facial appearance contributes to misgendering, social stigma, and/or threatens patient safety.

Patient readiness for surgery should also be considered in the context of pre-existing medical and psychiatric conditions. The authors recommend a thorough inquiry and documentation of past medical, surgical, and psychosocial history, active pharmacotherapies, and pertinent diagnostic tests. All comorbidities should be stable and well controlled, such that surgical risk is not unreasonably elevated. Although surgeons should always perform an independent assessment of each patient's operative risk, letters of support

(LOSs) from the patient's longitudinal mental health and primary care providers inform procedural clearance.

The physical examination is pivotal in determining which of the patient's facial features are discordant with their gender identity and ultimately informs procedural selection. To increase the likelihood of procedural coverage, surgeons should document their examination findings in a manner that explicitly and objectively substantiates the patient's gender incongruence. Specifically, facial features should be systematically and comprehensively analyzed, then recorded as imparting a masculinizing or feminizing appearance (**Fig. 1**).

Clinical photographs are another essential component of FGAS consultation that objectively supports the medical necessity of these procedures. As with all preoperative photographs, the patient should be positioned against a uniform, contrasting background and appropriately lit to minimize shadows. When capturing photographs for FGAS, it is also important to hold the patient's hair back with a hairband or headband, so their facial features and contour can be clearly and completely visualized. The photographer must take care to position the patient centrally and capture their hair, head, and neck in entirety—ideally using the clavicles to mark the inferior border of the frame. Distorting camera angles and features should be avoided. The patient should be captured in anterior-posterior, oblique, lateral, worm's-eye, and bird's-eye views.

The final step of FGAS consultation involves the surgeon's assessment and plan. Surgeons must consider the patient's goals and physical anatomy

to select which FGAS procedural components are medically necessary and feasible. The surgeon must then synthesize a list of planned procedures with corresponding common procedural terminology (CPT) codes. FGAS encompasses a subset of common CPT codes (**Fig. 2**); however, some insurance policies may not acknowledge certain codes. It is therefore imperative to carefully review each insurance carrier's utilization management guidelines prior to claim submission.[20]

Letters of Support

The SOC-8 requires patients seeking GAS to obtain one LOS from an independent qualified health care professional attesting to their candidacy for surgery.[12] However, prior versions of the SOC required two letters, one from a mental health professional and the other from a medical provider.[20] While most state and private insurers abide by the former recommendations, available research demonstrates that two opinions are largely unnecessary due to overwhelming correlation in provider opinion.[21] This requirement may evolve as policies are updated to reflect the current SOC, but two is the current accepted standard.

The mental health and medical LOS both contain pertinent patient history and diagnoses, certify medical necessity of FGAS, and attest to patient readiness for the surgery. While these letters are necessary to meet insurance requirements, they also inform surgeons' decision-making. Both letters must include basic information, such as the patient's legal and preferred

---

Physical Examination Documentation for Facial Feminization Surgery Consultation

"Top-down examination of the head and neck was performed, beginning with the upper facial third. The patient has a highly masculinized forehead contour, as evidenced by increased forehead length, clear frontal bossing from pneumatization of the frontal sinus, and temporal hollowing with prominent temporal ridges bilaterally. The hairline also lacks the typical contour that is commonly associated with a feminine face. Further, there is significant lateral orbital hooding secondary to prominence of the brow ridge and lateral orbital rims, which is highly stigmatic of a masculine face.

Examination of the middle facial third demonstrates a highly masculinized nasal profile, as evidenced by the patient's prominent dorsal nasal hump, wide and divergent nasal bones through the mid-vault, and acute nasolabial angle approximating 90 degrees. There is also a projected radix due to pneumatization of the frontal sinus that further exacerbates the patient's clearly masculine facial form. In addition, malar prominences lack the typical volume and softness that is commonly seen in the feminine face. The cutaneous upper lip length is increased with lack of vermilion height and show, which is also a highly masculinizing facial feature.

Examination of the lower facial third also demonstrates highly masculinizing features, including: wide gonial prominences, an angular and wide central chin, and square lower jaw contour. Overall chin position is anterior relative to the anterior facial plane when viewed laterally, which also imparts a masculine contour to the face.

Examination of the neck demonstrates prominence of the thyroid cartilage which is characteristically a stigmatic masculine feature."

Fig. 1. Sample documentation of examination findings during the facial feminization surgery consultation, which frame the patient's facial characteristics as highly stigmatic and masculinizing. (*Courtesy of* R. Ettinger, MD, Seattle, WA.)

Common Procedural Terminology Codes for Facial Gender Affirming Surgery	
Upper Facial Third	
67900	Browlift mid-forehead or coronal approach
14020	Adjacent tissue transfer of scalp – 10 sq cm or less
14021	Adjacent tissue transfer of scalp – 10.1 sq cm to 30 sq cm
21139	Frontal sinus setback
21209	Osteoplasty, orbital rim contouring
67950	Canthoplasty
Middle Facial Third	
30400	Rhinoplasty-primary, lateral and alar cartilages and elevation of nasal tip
30410	Rhinoplasty-complete, external parts including bony pyramid
30420	Primary septorhinoplasty, including major septal repair
14061	Adjacent tissue transfer of lips – 10 sq cm or less
Lower Facial Third & Neck	
21121	Genioplasty, sliding single piece
21122	Genioplasty, sliding, two or more osteotomies for asymmetrical chin or bone wedge reversal for asymmetrical chin
21123	Genioplasty, sliding, augmentation with interpositional bone grafts, includes obtaining bone grafts
21209-22	Osteoplasty, mandibular contouring, this is a separate and distinct surgical site accessed through a transoral mucosal incision that increases the complexity of the case, and increases the surgical time by great than 1 hour
31599	Chondrolaryngoplasty
General	
15773	Fat grafting, to face, eyelids, mouth 25cc or less
15774	Fat grafting, to face, eyelids, mouth, each additional 25cc of injectate
64646	Botox injection, such as for masseteric muscle hypertrophy

Fig. 2. Summary of pertinent facial gender-affirming surgery common procedural terminology codes for procedural authorization. (*Courtesy of* R. Ettinger, MD, Seattle, WA.)

names, gender identity, preferred pronouns, and date of birth. Letter writers should include the date of evaluation, their license or credentials, and detail the duration and nature of their relationship with the patient. Each letter should confirm the patient's persistent gender incongruence between assigned sex at birth and gender identity, including the date of social transition if applicable. Letter writers must explicitly confirm the patient's diagnosis of gender dysphoria (ICD-10 F64.1) and indicate that the patient's gender dysphoria causes clinically significant distress or impairment. Prior gender-affirming treatments, such as mental health support, hormone therapy, and prior surgical procedures, should also be included. Further, both letter writers should support the patient's candidacy for facial feminization or masculinization surgery. Finally, a handwritten "wet" signature is required, as insurers consider digital signatures to be invalid.[22]

The primary distinction between the medical and mental health clearance letters involves provider type and review of co-existing diagnoses. The mental health LOS should focus on psychosocial conditions, such as mental health diagnoses—including substance use, corresponding treatments, and social supports. Qualified professionals include psychiatrists (MD, DO), psychologists (MA,

PhD, PsyD), psychiatric nurse practitioners (ARNP, PMHNP), licensed marriage and family therapists, licensed independent clinical social workers, and mental health counselors. In contrast, the medical clearance letter is typically from a medically focused professional, such as a primary care physician or advanced practice provider. The medical LOS is expected to summarize pertinent medical and surgical history, medications, and social history. If the medical letter writer is involved in treating the patient's mental health conditions, the provider may also comment on related psychiatric diagnoses and interventions. Both providers must attest that co-existing conditions are stable, well controlled, and will not contribute to undue surgical risk. The sample LOS template in **Fig. 3** exemplifies essential content for each LOS, as well as differences between the mental health and medical clearance letters.[22]

Preoperative Insurance Authorization

The insurance authorization process for FGAS is complex and highly variable based on insurance carrier, plan benefits, and geographic location. It is essential to collect all necessary documentation with meticulous attention to each insurer's requirements prior to initiating the authorization process.

Sample Letter of Support Template

[Institutional Letterhead] [Date]
Re: [patient name on insurance card], [patient's chosen name], [patient DOB]

Dear Doctor,

[Patient name] is a patient in my care at [practice name] since [date]. [Patient name] identifies as [gender identity] and goes by [pronouns] pronouns. [Patient name] first knew [pronoun] gender identity differed from [pronoun] assigned sex at age [age]. [Patient name] has successfully socially transitioned by [list how – name, pronouns, dress, hair etc.] [Patient name] has consistently lived in a gender role congruent with [pronoun] affirmed gender since [date]. [Patient name] has consistently been on hormone therapy since [date] (if contraindicated or chosen not to take hormones, state here). Despite these interventions, [pronoun] reports persistent anxiety, depression, and distress related to [pronoun] gender incongruence. I conducted an independent evaluation of [patient name] and diagnosed [pronoun] with clinically significant and sustained Gender Dysphoria (ICD-10 F64.1).

[Pronoun] has expressed a persistent desire for [procedure name]. [Pronoun] goals of surgery are [goals]. Surgery will address [pronoun] gender dysphoria in these ways: [explain].

USE FOR MEDICAL CLEARANCE ONLY:
A complete medical evaluation was performed. [Patient name] has the following co-existing medical conditions: [list of diagnoses], which are adequately managed by [list interventions]. [Pronoun]'s surgical history includes: [surgical history]. [Patient name] has no issues with illicit drug use and [pronoun] are stably housed (if untrue, explain stabilization plan). I see no present or uncontrolled medical or psychosocial conditions that would contradict surgical readiness.

USE FOR MENTAL HEALTH CLEARANCE ONLY:
A complete psychosocial evaluation was performed. [Patient name] has the following co-existing behavioral health conditions: [list of diagnoses], which are adequately managed by [list interventions]. [Patient name] has no issues with illicit drug use and [pronoun] are stably housed (if untrue, explain stabilization plan). I see no present or uncontrolled psychosocial conditions that would contradict surgical readiness.

[Patient name] has more than met the WPATH criteria for [procedure name] and has an excellent understanding surgical risks, benefits, and alternatives. [Patient name] is capable of making an informed decision about surgery and prepared for post-operative recovery. I believe the next appropriate step for [pronoun] is to undergo [procedure name], which will help in further treating [pronoun] gender dysphoria. I hereby recommend and refer [patient name] to have this surgery. If you have any questions or concerns, please do not hesitate to contact myself or my office.

Sincerely,

[Provider handwritten signature]
[Provider name, credentials]
[Provider location, phone number]

Fig. 3. Sample letter of support template for medical or mental health clearance. (*Adapted from* publicly available templates created by The University of Washington Transgender and Gender Non-Binary Health Program, Seattle, WA.[22])

As previously stated, this includes surgeon consultation, medical and mental health LOS, proposed CPT codes, and, in some cases, patient photographs. This process often requires advocacy from the patient, physician, and administrative support staff. It is therefore essential for all multidisciplinary team members to be familiar with common insurance terminology and procedures to circumnavigate denials.

Two pertinent terms to understand and differentiate are prior authorization and predetermination. Prior authorization, also known as preauthorization or precertification, is the process by which patient eligibility and medical necessity for a given procedure is determined preoperatively. In contrast, predetermination refers to preoperative review of the patient's benefits to ascertain if the proposed procedure is covered by their insurance plan.

Obtaining prior authorization independent of predetermination, or vice versa, does not guarantee coverage or reimbursement of procedural cost. For example, a surgeon may perform a procedure based on successful preauthorization, but lack of benefit coverage may result in the claim being partially or fully denied—despite medical necessity. It is also important to note that neither prior authorization nor predetermination are legally required; thus, some insurers do not offer these services. However, when available, it is imperative for the surgical team to obtain both prior authorization and predetermination to ensure appropriate reimbursement.[20]

Another important concept is in-network versus out-of-network, which describes coverage and reimbursement relationships between surgeons and insurers. In-network physicians and practices are contracted to provide services at a negotiated rate through specific insurance carriers. As a result, insurers often cover a greater percentage of incurred in-network health care costs, which translates to cost-savings for patients and easier claims processes for providers. Conversely, out-of-network surgeon services are more expensive and may be partially or completely denied by insurers, placing disproportionate financial burden on patients.[20]

It may be beneficial for surgeons to obtain a single case agreement or letter of agreement, which refers to pre-agreed upon coverage for a particular set of procedures, including CPT codes and corresponding reimbursement. Single case agreements are difficult to obtain, but compulsory for out-of-network surgeons, as they protect physicians and patients from financial liability. However, single case agreements should also be considered by in-network providers. Although this request is atypical for most in-network procedures, FGAS CPT codes are often unlisted and lack standardization. Single case agreements therefore offer in-network physicians more defined coverage and reimbursement.[20]

Similar to single case agreements, carve-out agreements involve predetermined coverage and reimbursement of a defined set of CPT codes. Unlike single case agreements, which are determined on a patient-by-patient basis, carve-out agreements are umbrella policies that apply to all patients under the care of involved providers and insurers. Carve-out agreements are ideal for high-volume FGAS surgeons, as these policies reduce the administrative burden for practices and insurers.[20]

Postoperative Insurance Claim Submission

Insurance claim submission is the process by which health care providers request payment for services rendered to patients. Claim submission protocol differs by practice but commonly involves claim preparation by the billing department or administrative staff. Claims include supporting documents that illustrate procedural necessity and execution, such as surgeon consultation and operative notes and preauthorization, predetermination, or single case agreement details. Administrators also often confirm CPT codes to ensure accuracy and consistency across health care claims prior to submission. Claims may then be sent to insurers electronically or manually using 1 of 2 forms: (1) CMS-1500, which is used for noninstitutional health care facilities, or (2) UB-04, which is a variation of the CMS-1500 form that is used for institutional health care

facilities such as hospitals. Once submitted, insurers review the claim for accuracy and verify that the services provided are covered under the patient's insurance plan.[20,23,24]

Addressing Barriers to Insurance Approval

Successful insurance authorization and reimbursement for FGAS is a formidable process that may be slowed by a failure to meet insurance requirements and/or coverage limitations. While there are many measures that providers and administrators can take to optimize procedural coverage, even the most experienced team may encounter partial or complete denials.

First and foremost, the importance of specialized administrative and clinical support teams dedicated to GAS cannot be understated. As FGAS often requires extensive peri-operative coordination, knowledgeable team members optimize efficiency, communication, and patient outcomes. This should involve timely appointment scheduling, preoperative and postoperative education and assessments, communication with ancillary providers, and interactions with insurance companies, including preparation of claims. This support reduces both patient and physician stress and administrative burden.

With respect to documentation, it may be difficult for even the most experienced FGAS providers to consistently fulfill the exhaustive criteria mandated by insurers. As such, the authors strongly recommend the use of templated notes with modifiable statements addressing salient history and examination points (see **Figs. 1** and **3**). This strategy minimizes variabilities in verbiage and data collection, thereby reducing potential for claim denials.

When discrepancies or omissions arise, insurance companies will request clarifying documentation from providers. For example, during prior authorization and predetermination, insurers may ask physicians to justify CPT codes or anticipated length of stay by writing a letter of medical necessity. Such formalities create an additional administrative burden on providers but are imperative in fulfilling insurance requirements.

In some instances, insurance policies have exclusionary clauses that prohibit coverage of one or more specific components of the proposed FGAS procedures. These coverage gaps present unfortunate and challenging obstacles for patients and physicians. In these scenarios, a formal policy review should be conducted to understand the nuances of the insurance policy in question. When certain treatments are not explicitly covered, alternative treatments should be considered. If no alternatives exist and a formal denial has been issued, an appeal may be submitted.

Denials may occur at any point after prior authorization or claim submission. Patients and physicians have the right to appeal each denial, should they so choose. Although appeal processes vary by insurer, most companies require a formal statement from the petitioner stating the medical necessity of the denied procedure and the desired action resulting from the appeal. Appeals are first reviewed internally by the insurance company to affirm the validity of the denial.[25] If the internal appeal is unsuccessful, an external appeal may be undertaken. This process involves an impartial review of the denial by an unaffiliated third-party or independent review organization, who will affirm or overturn the denial.[26] This is an important feature of the appeal process that limits bias and inequity.

SUMMARY

In summary, the FGAS consultation, documentation, and insurance authorization processes are complex and riddled with administrative and legal obstacles. Surgeons, ancillary providers, and affiliated team members must be experienced in these practices to obtain insurance approvals for FGAS procedures without delay or exception. This ultimately improves equity and access to medically necessary care for the TGD population.

CLINICS CARE POINTS

- Facial GAS is a critical component of TGD health care that is strongly associated with psychosocial and quality of life benefits due to improvements in both self-perception and public perception, yet these surgeries are less likely to be acknowledged or reimbursed by insurers than body-affirming procedures.

- Gender incongruence is defined as an incompatibility between an individual's psychological sense of gender and their assigned sex at birth. While gender incongruence is a component of insurance criteria, a diagnosis of persistent, well-documented gender dysphoria—or distress related to one's gender incongruence—is the crux of most policies.

- Surgeons must meticulously document all aspects of their preoperative consultation to affirm (1) the patient's diagnosis of gender dysphoria and (2) the medical necessity of the proposed procedure.

- Most insurers require 2 LOSs from independent qualified mental health and medical professionals attesting to the patient's persistent, sustained gender dysphoria and candidacy for the surgery.

- Prior authorization and predetermination are important components of the preoperative insurance process that address procedural medical necessity and benefit coverage, respectively, and ultimately facilitate transparency between patients, providers, and payers.

- In-network physicians are contracted to provide services at a negotiated rate through specific insurance carriers, resulting in cost-savings for patients and reliable reimbursements for providers.

- Lack of standardization in medical coding for facial GAS negatively impacts patient cost-burden and physician reimbursement. Single case and carve-out agreements, which involve predetermined coverage and reimbursement of a defined set of CPT codes, help to minimize financial liability of patients and providers.

- Patients and providers have a right to appeal insurance denials by means of internal and external reviews. External third-party involvement reduces bias in the claim denial process.

DISCLOSURE

The authors have no relevant or material financial interests that relate to the research and sources described in this article.

REFERENCES

1. Jody H, Andrew F, Kathryn O. How many adults and youth identify as transgender in the United States? Los Angeles, CA: The Williams Institute; 2022. Available at: https://williamsinstitute.law.ucla.edu/publications/trans-adults-united-states/. Accessed November 10, 2023.
2. James SE, Herman JL, Rankin S, et al. The report of the 2015 U.S. transgender survey. Washington, DC: National Center for Transgender Equality; 2016. Available at: https://transequality.org/sites/default/files/docs/usts/USTS-Full-Report-Dec17.pdf. Accessed November 18, 2023.
3. Wiegmann AL, Young EI, Baker KE, et al. The affordable care act and its impact on plastic and gender-affirmation surgery. Plast Reconstr Surg 2021;147:135–53.
4. Gorbea E, Gidumal S, Kozato A, et al. Insurance coverage of facial gender affirmation surgery: A

review of Medicaid and commercial insurance. Oto-laryngol Head Neck Surg 2021;165(6):791–7.

5. Bakko M, Kattari SK. Transgender-related insurance denials as barriers to transgender healthcare: Differences in experience by insurance type. J Gen Intern Med 2020;35(6):1693–700.

6. Trans Legislation Tracker 2022. Available at: https://translegislation.com/bills/2022. Accessed November 13, 2023.

7. Chou DW, Bruss D, Tejani N, et al. Quality of life outcomes after facial feminization surgery. Facial Plast Surg Aesthet Med 2022;24(S2). S-44-S-46.

8. Gulati A, Zebolsky A, Patel N, et al. Satisfaction and quality of life following gender-affirming facial surgery. Facial Plast Surg Aesthet Med 2023;25(4):355–7.

9. Siringo NV, Berman ZP, Boczar D, et al. Techniques and trends of facial feminization surgery: a systematic review and representative case report. Ann Plast Surg 2022;88(6):704–11.

10. Hauc SC, Mateja KL, Long AS, et al. Limited access to facial feminization geographically despite nationwide expansion of other gender-affirming surgeries. Plast Reconstr Surg Glob Open 2022;10(9):e4521.

11. Standards of Care History and Purpose. World Professional Association for Transgender Health. Available at: https://www.wpath.org/soc8/history. Accessed November 10, 2023.

12. Coleman E, Radix AE, Bouman WP, et al. Standards of Care for the health of transgender and gender diverse people, version 8. Int J Transgend Health 2022;23:S1–259.

13. Diaddigo SE, Lavalley MN, Asadourian PA, et al. Concordance of national insurance criteria with WPATH Standards of Care for gender-affirming surgery. Plast Reconstr Surg 2023. https://doi.org/10.1097/PRS.0000000000011144. Online ahead of print.

14. Becker I, Auer M, Barkmann C, et al. A cross-sectional multicenter study of multidimensional body image in adolescents and adults with gender dysphoria before and after transition-related medical interventions. Arch Sex Behav 2018;47(8):2335–47.

15. El-Hadi H, Stone J, Temple-Oberle C, et al. Gender-affirming surgery for transgender individuals: Perceived satisfaction and barriers to care. Plas Surg 2018;26(4):263–8.

16. Staples JM, Bird ER, Gregg JJ, et al. Improving the gender-affirmation process for transgender and gender-nonconforming individuals: Associations among time since transition began, body satisfaction, and sexual distress. J Sex Res 2020;57(3):375–83.

17. Wiepjes CM, Nota NM, de Blok CJM, et al. The Amsterdam cohort of gender dysphoria study (1972-2015): Trends in prevalence, treatment, and regrets. J Sex Med 2018;15(4):582–90.

18. Diagnostic and statistical manual of mental disorders. 5th edition. American Psychiatric Association; 2022. Text Revision (DSM-5-TR).

19. Gender incongruence and transgender health in the ICD. World Health Organization. Available at: https://www.who.int/standards/classifications/frequently-asked-questions/gender-incongruence-and-transgender-health-in-the-icd. Accessed November 12, 2023.

20. Kuperstock JE. Getting to yes: Navigating the insurance gauntlet. Facial Plast Surg Clin N Am 2023;31:371–4.

21. Jones BA, Brewin N, Richards C, et al. Investigating the outcome of the initial assessment at a national transgender health service: Time to review the process? Int J Transgenderism 2017;18(4):427–32.

22. Gender affirming care at UW Medicine. University of Washington Transgender and Nonbinary Health Program. Available at: https://depts.washington.edu/tgnb. Accessed November 18, 2023.

23. More about insurance and insurance claims processing. Medical Billing and Coding Certification. Available at: https://www.medicalbillingandcoding.org/insurance-claims-process/. Accessed November 22, 2023.

24. Electronic billing. Center for Medicare and Medicaid Services. Available at: https://www.cms.gov/medicare/coding-billing/electronic-billing. Accessed November 22, 2023.

25. Appealing a health plan decision. Healthcare.gov. Available at: https://www.healthcare.gov/appeal-insurance-company-decision/. Accessed November 22, 2023.

26. Appeals process. Premera Blue Cross. Available at: https://www.premera.com/documents/019804.pdf. Accessed November 22, 2023.

Preoperative Radiology and Virtual Surgical Planning

Brendan J. Cronin, MD*, Justine C. Lee, MD, PhD

KEYWORDS

- Preoperative radiology • Virtual surgical planning • Facial gender affirming surgery
- Facial feminization surgery • Facial masculinization surgery

KEY POINTS

- Key regions of the face manipulated with virtual surgical planning include the nasofrontal complex, superolateral orbit, mandible, and chin.
- Preoperative clinical facial analysis coupled with patient-specific triggers of dysphoria is key for operative planning and postoperative patient satisfaction.
- In FFS, osseus maneuvers are targeted toward bony reduction while in FMS, implants, augmentation, or genioplasty techniques target skeletal augmentation.
- Use of 3D technology to compare patient and standardized anatomic reference skulls provides objective metrics for planning osseus movements.
- VSP has been shown to decrease dural violation and nerve injury and improve operative efficiency. Future comparative cohort studies are needed to examine patient-reported outcomes in FGAS with and without VSP.

INTRODUCTION

Background

In facial gender affirming surgery (FGAS), precise and meticulous preoperative planning plays a pivotal role. The importance of this planning derives from the objective of FGAS to transform native preoperative anatomy to that of a different masculine/feminine appearance, as opposed to restoring normal from abnormal form in congenital anomalies or traumatic craniofacial injuries. In particular, bony movements and osteotomies lie at the crux craniofacial skeletal transformation, upon which are manipulated features of the soft tissue envelope.[1–3]

Various preoperative planning techniques and intraoperative 'guides'' have been employed in determining the optimal location of osteotomies for FGAS. These methods encompass a range of approaches, including transillumination of the frontal sinus during perioperative clinical examination,[4] preoperative evaluation of sinus dimensions through radiographs[5] or computed tomography (CT) scans,[6,7] utilization of measurements from various anthropometric landmarks,[1] intraoperative assessment solely based on the surgeon's experience without preoperative imaging,[8,9] implementing three-dimensional (3D) printing of patient skulls to simulate maneuvers before the actual surgery,[10,11] and utilizing 3D photogrammetry for planning. Despite these advancements, certain osseous maneuvers like frontal setback, reduction genioplasty, and gonial angle reduction were traditionally performed free-hand after being planned using the aforementioned methods. Similarly, in facial masculinization surgery (FMS), augmentation of the craniofacial skeleton was performed using methyl methacrylate or calcium hydroxyapatite constructs, as well as onlay bone grafting. The advent of virtual surgical planning (VSP) and its

Division of Plastic and Reconstructive Surgery, University of California, Los Angeles, 200 Medical Plaza, Suite 460, Los Angeles, CA 90095, USA
* Corresponding author.
E-mail address: BCronin@mednet.ucla.edu

Oral Maxillofacial Surg Clin N Am 36 (2024) 171–182
https://doi.org/10.1016/j.coms.2023.12.006
1042-3699/24/© 2023 Elsevier Inc. All rights reserved.

widespread application in pediatric craniofacial and orthognathic surgery marked the transition to guide-directed osteotomies[12,13] and custom implants, which were then adopted in the growing field of FGAS.

Indications

The use of VSP in FGAS has been a topic of debate.[2,8–11,14] Some authors caution against employing VSP, arguing that a 'color by number' approach might lead to a standardized process disregarding individualized anatomy and esthetic considerations.[8,9] Additionally, they express concerns that relying on VSP could reduce the surgeon's role to that of a technician merely following predetermined guides, hindering learning and creativity.[8,9]

In comparison, several authors have reported using some form of computer-aided planning for FGAS,[2,10,14] and one group even developed specialized VSP software tailored for FGAS procedures.[10]

In our practice, we believe VSP improves intraoperative precision, safety, and speed of all skeletal movements. As a result, we obtain a preoperative maxillofacial CT with 0.6 mm cuts for surgical planning and VSP for all patients. Decision making during the VSP session is based on clinical examination, cephalometric measurements, and comparison to a reference female skull.[15] While there are no specific contraindications to the use of VSP, its cost and the cost of custom guide/implant manufacturing may limit availability depending on practice setting and institution.

PREOPERATIVE CLINICAL EVALUATION AND RADIOGRAPHIC PLANNING FOR VIRTUAL SURGICAL PLANNING

The key anatomic considerations in FGAS center around the differences between the male and female facial skeleton and soft tissues.[1,16] **Table 1** provides a review of these key anatomic differences. Examination of the patient—both clinical and radiographic—inform VSP and operative planning. Key features are outlined in the following paragraphs.

Clinical Examination

The clinical assessment encompasses several key aspects, which are shown in **Fig. 1**. To begin, the position, shape, and any temporal recession of the hairline are carefully examined. Moving to the forehead, the length at the midline and above the lateral brow, along with eyebrow position and symmetry, are considered. The frontal bone is then assessed, observing lateral orbital hooding in the frontal view and supraorbital bossing and nasofrontal complex contour in the lateral view.

The mandible is analyzed focusing on the gonial angle, gonial flaring, lower facial width, and dental occlusion. The chin is also thoroughly evaluated for its length, height, and projection. Lip length and the upper white lip to red lip ratio are examined, as well as performing a comprehensive analysis of the entire nose.

Radiographic Workup

We obtain fine-cut maxillofacial CT (section thickness of 0.6 mm) and 3D reconstruction in all patients undergoing FGAS for virtual planning. We assess these scans for evaluation of the (1) nasofrontal complex, (2) mandible, and (3) chin. In the upper third of the face (1), we evaluate forehead type (**Table 2**),[1] frontal sinus size and dimensions, anterior table thickness, sagittal distance between the anterior-most portion of the globe and the frontal bone on sagittal view, and nasofrontal angle. In the mandible (2), we assess bigonial width, gonial flaring, and gonial angle/mandibular height (**Fig. 2**). Regarding the chin (3), we analyze upper facial height to lower facial height ratio and the Holdaway ratio to determine the need for and magnitude of chin reposition, reduction, or augmentation (**Fig. 3**). We also examine the course of the inferior alveolar nerve and map its proximity to any planned gonial angle reduction/ostectomy or genioplasty osteotomies. Relationships of the maxilla and mandible to each other and the skull base are also examined to reveal any underlying skeletal discrepancies or malocclusion that would indicate the need for orthognathic surgery (if necessary, this is performed prior to all other feminization procedures as a separate surgery).

Virtual Surgical Planning

Preoperative planning of the osseous maneuvers of FGAS is performed using a standard female or male skull as a reference. 3D CT scans of a representative patient's skull and the skull of a reference female are shown (**Fig. 4**).

These reconstructions are subsequently superimposed to identify the precise areas of modification of the underlying craniofacial skeleton (**Fig. 5**). For FFS, these include reduction at the forehead (red dotted line), gonial angles (blue dotted line), and chin (yellow dotted line) (see **Fig. 4**). For FMS, this includes an estimate on the increased bigonial width, mandibular height, gonial angle, chin height, and width and projection required for skeletal masculinization (see **Fig. 2**). The reference skull (see **Fig. 5**; orange 'mask') is scaled relative to the patient skull (white 'mask'), and aligned in the vertical and horizontal planes. The images are 'zeroed' and the volumetric difference

Table 1
Differences in male/female facial characteristics

Characteristic	Male	Female
Frontal bone	• Larger, broader frontal bone • Larger frontal sinus • Flat and retroclined frontal bone on lateral view	• Smaller frontal bone • Smaller frontal sinus • Gentle curve from frontonasal junction to hairline on lateral view
Orbits	• Prominent supraorbital bossing/lateral orbital hooding	• No supraorbital bossing/lateral orbital hooding
Zygoma	• Flatter, lower, and less prominent zygomatic arch	• Higher and more projecting zygomas
Mandible	• Wider lower facial width • Acute gonial angle	• Narrower lower facial width • Gentler, less-defined gonial angle
Chin	• Wider and 'boxier' chin with increased height and projection	• Narrow, pointed chin, generally shorter and less projected
Forehead Hairline Brow	• Higher 'M' shaped hairline with bitemporal recession • Flatter brows that sit lower across the orbital ridge	• Lower 'O' shaped hairline without recession • Curved brows that arch above the supraorbital rims
Nose	• Larger nose with acute glabellar and nasolabial angles • Prominent dorsal hump or straight dorsum	• Smaller nose with more obtuse nasolabial and glabellar angles • Narrower with possible concavity or supratip break
Lips	• Longer and thinner lips • Minimal incisal show in repose	• Fuller and shorter lips with increased visibility of the vermilion • Greater incisal show in repose

between the patient and reference skull is mapped (green). Surgical maneuvers to correct discrepant skeletal areas between the patient and reference skull are then planned virtually (**Fig. 6**). VSP services are provided by 3D Systems (Rock Hill, SC)

CUTTING GUIDES AND CUSTOM IMPLANTS

Various custom cutting guides, implants, and management algorithms for both FFS and FMS are shown (**Figs. 7–13**).

OPERATIVE TECHNIQUE
Facial Feminization Surgery

Frontal setback
Type III foreheads In type III foreheads, we generate a custom cutting guide that incorporates both a frontal sinus osteotomy guide and a 'porcupine guide.' After appropriate exposure, this guide is positioned on the frontal bone by footplates that extend into the superior orbital rims. The specific anatomy of these footplates allows facile and accurate positioning of the custom 3D-printed guide.

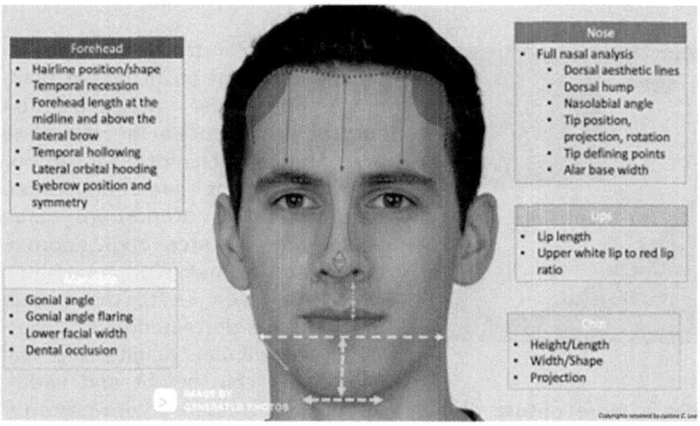

Fig. 1. Clinical examination and facial analysis. An overview of elements of facial analysis is demonstrated and annotated. A systematic and reproducible method of clinical examination ensures all elements of facial esthetics are taken into consideration during consultation. Key characteristics to evaluate for VSP include forehead contour and supraorbital bossing, lower facial width with gonial angle severity, and chin position, width, and projection. (*From* Photograph provided by www.generated.photos, an open-access platform using AI software to generate realistic human portraits.)

Table 2
Ousterhout classification of forehead types

Forehead Type	Features	Management
Type I	• Mild bossing, no or minimum frontal sinus • Thick anterior wall	• Burring
Type II	• Moderate bossing, midforehead flattening • Normal forehead protrusion	• Burring plus cement filling
Type III	• Significant bossing, large projection • Large frontal sinus with thin anterior table	• Anterior frontal sinus wall setback
Type IV	• Severe forehead slope not amenable to setback	• Cement filling to create esthetic forehead profile without setback

The outline of the frontal sinus osteotomy is marked with a bone pencil or bonny blue dye, and a 2.7 mm drill guide and 2.7 mm drill are used to drill into the frontal bone at varying depths based on the guide. The holes are infiltrated with dye to clearly demonstrate depth of the desired reduction. The cutting guide is removed and oblique osteotomies performed to remove the anterior table. The frontal bone is then recontoured on the back table to achieve the preplanned setback. A pineapple burr is then used to recontour the forehead, superior orbital rims, and lateral orbital rims. Certain custom cutting guides may also incorporate planned ostectomies of the superolateral orbit, which are marked and carried out in a similar fashion as discussed earlier. Otherwise, these areas are reduced via burring. The radix is also burred to ensure a smooth transition to the anterior table of the frontal sinus. The anterior table of the frontal sinus is then replaced and secured with plates and screws.

Type I foreheads In these patients, absence of the frontal sinus or sufficient thickness of the anterior table with mild supraorbital bossing permits frontal recontouring with burring alone without osteotomy. A porcupine guide is seated on the exposed

forehead via footplates into the orbit and secured with 5 mm screws. A similar aforementioned process is followed and the forehead and orbits recontoured with a rotating pineapple burr.

Gonial angle reduction
Gonial angle reduction can be achieved through ostectomy or burring. In cases of ostectomy, cutting guides are positioned based on splints of the mandibular dentition or the contours of the ascending ramus and secured with 4 mm screws. A disadvantage of this approach is that either type of guide requires wide mucosal incision and subperiosteal exposure for seating of the guide and adequate visualization/maneuvering during ostectomy. Ostectomy is then performed with a reciprocating saw, ultrasonic saw, or side-cutting saw, depending on surgeon preference. As a tradeoff for extensive exposure and periosteal denuding, ostectomy yields bone segments that can be used as an interposition bone graft to buttress a concomitant genioplasty. If achieving reduction through burring, smaller mucosal incisions, wide enough only for the passage of a protected oscillating power rasp and channel retractor, can be used. Reduction is guided by a VSP-generated heat map of the mandibular contours indicating

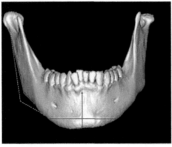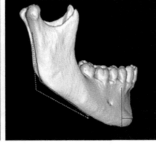

Fig. 2. 3D reconstruction of an assigned female at birth patient planning for facial masculinization surgery. Differences in masculine and feminine craniofacial contour and dimensions are highlighted (*red* = female proportions, *blue dotted line* indicates rough approximation of a masculine mandible). On frontal view (*left*), the female mandible has decreased vertical posterior mandibular height, bigonial width, and chin height and width. On lateral view, the female mandible has a more obtuse gonial angle and decreased antero-posterior chin projection.

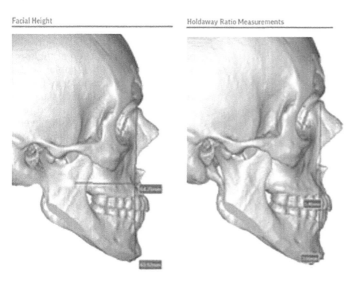

Fig. 3. Dentofacial analysis and cephalometric ratios in VSP. Orthognathic and dentofacial analysis ratios, including the facial height and Holdaway ratio, are mapped preoperatively to guide operative maneuvers. Facial height (distance from glabella to menton) is used to calculate the ratio of upper (glabella to subnasale) and lower (subnasale to menton) facial height and informs the need for vertical chin repositioning. Holdaway ratio is defined by the ratio of (1) the horizontal distance from vertical plane NB to the anterior-most aspect of the lower incisor (NB-LI) and (2) the horizontal distance from vertical plane NB to the anterior-most aspect of the bony chin or pogonion (NB-Po). This ratio informs the need for chin repositioning in the horizontal plane (sliding genioplasty). Above, an NB-LI of 5.46 mm and NB-Po of 3.66 yields a Holdaway ratio of 1.5, indicating the need for chin advancement. (*Courtesy of* Justine C. Lee, MD, PhD, California, USA.)

the degree of reduction in millimeters of various regions. Commonly, the final reduction of the inferior-most aspect of the mandibular border is performed by palpation alone. In the appropriately selected patient, we find rasping alone tends to better preserve soft tissue draping and limit postoperative jowling.

Reduction genioplasty

VSP plans for genioplasty are incumbent upon patient-specific preoperative anatomy and may incorporate reduction or augmentation of chin height, chin advancement, and chin narrowing. We perform genioplasty in any patient who requires advancement, narrowing, or an increase in vertical height. Less severe phenotypes or those with excessively wide or prominent chins can be managed with burring alone.

VSP for genioplasty, in particular, enables highly specific transfer of operative plans to the operative field by guiding bone cuts (osteotomy guides) and exact relationships of bony segments

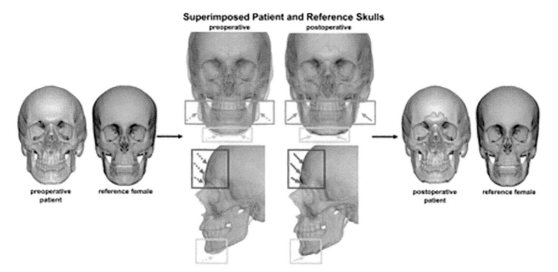

Fig. 4. Simulation of Osseus reduction of the nasofrontal complex and lower third of the face as derived from reference anatomic model skulls. 3D reconstructions of the patient's craniofacial skeleton and a 3D reconstruction of a 'model' feminine skull are overlapped and areas of nasofrontal (*red arrows*), mandibular (*blue arrows*), and chin excess (*yellow arrows*) identified. These are virtually reduced to yield the 3D model representing the final surgical goal from which cutting and contour guides are derived.

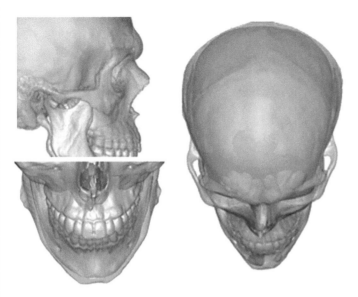

Fig. 5. Modeling osseous maneuvers on a female skull. Superimposed reference and patient skulls identify the precise areas of reduction at the forehead (*red dotted line*), gonial angles (*blue dotted line*), and chin (*yellow dotted line*). The reference skull (see Fig. 3B; *orange* 'mask') is scaled relative to the patient skull (*white* 'mask') based on the position of the nasion and overlap of the anterior aspect of the maxilla and zygomatic arches. Vertical position is set via alignment of the infraorbital rims and apex of the skull. Horizontal position is set based on symmetry of the zygomatic arches. The images are 'zeroed' and the volumetric difference between the patient and reference skull is mapped (*green*). (*Courtesy of* Justine C. Lee, MD, PhD, California, USA.)

on fixation (custom prefabricated plates). In patients with significant masculine features, our approach involves a reduction genioplasty. This technique consists of a horizontal osteotomy accompanied by a central vertical wedge resection of the chin segment, performed with a reciprocating saw guided by prefabricated cutting guides. The bony segments are then secured with the custom titanium plate using predrilled holes. Recontouring of the inferior mandibular border after advancement may be required to smoothen any bony step offs.

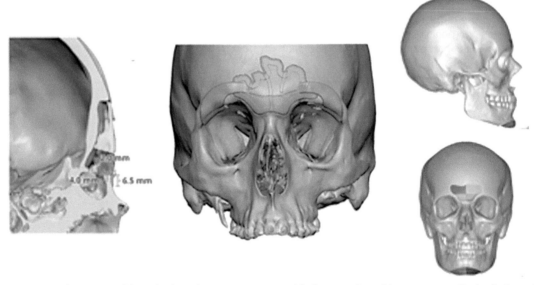

Fig. 6. VSP of anterior table setback and custom cutting guide for anterior table osteotomy. Sagittal view of planned anterior table setback (*left*) with frontal bone segments (*navy blue, light blue*) in their planned setback position. The degree of setback (2.0 mm), anterior table thickness (4.0 mm), and extent of frontal bone to the nasion/nasofrontal suture (6.5 mm) are planned preoperatively. The frontal bone that will be burred separately from the anterior table setback is show in green. The osteotomy guide is shown in orange (*right*). Our custom guide for the forehead setback includes a cutting edge around the periphery of the frontal sinus—osteotomies are designed to be made at the outer edge of the guide. This design leaves an appropriate rim of cortical bone at the periphery of the bone flap so that the flap does not 'fall into' the widened sinus when replaced after burring. (*Courtesy of* Justine C. Lee, MD, PhD, California, USA.)

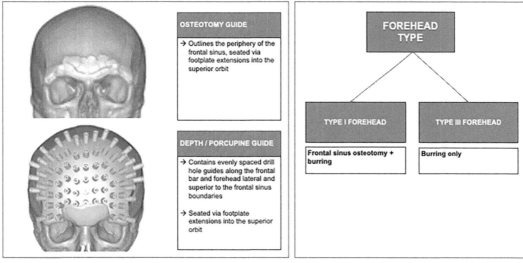

Fig. 7. Custom guides and algorithm for forehead setback (FFS).

In patients with less masculine chin phenotypes, guide-directed recontouring is performed. A dentition-registered guide is seated and the chin is drilled and marked with Bonney blue dye in a process similar to the forehead setback. Rasping with an oscillating power rasp as guided by the drilled and dye-stained holes is then performed until adequate reduction is achieved.

Facial Masculinization Surgery

Forehead augmentation is rare in clinical practice. In reality, most FMS procedures focus on augmenting the dimensions of the lower third of the face per patient requests.

Gonial angle augmentation

Augmentation of the gonial angle has been described using alloplastic materials such as silicone and porous polyethylene implants as well as more invasive autologous techniques involving placement of bone graft between a sagittal split osteotomy of the ramus and in the belly of the masseter muscle.[2,17,18]

We perform gonial angle augmentation using custom-fabricated porous polyethylene implants (Stryker, Kalamazoo, MI). The design is tailored to facial cephalometrics and patient preferences. Specifically, the desired vertical mandibular height, gonial angle definition, and gonial angle width are planned (see **Fig. 4**). Given the degree

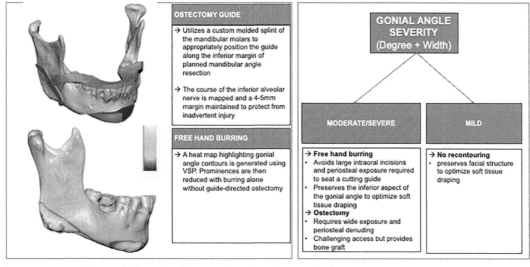

Fig. 8. Custom guides and algorithm for gonial angle reduction (FFS).

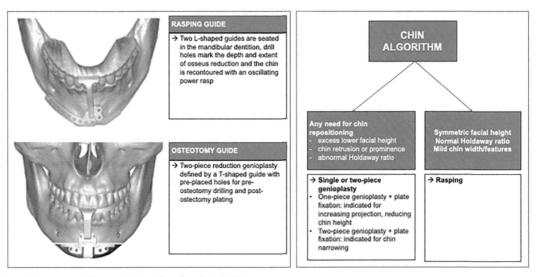

Fig. 9. Custom guides and algorithm for chin (FFS).

of augmentation typically desired and the need to access the inferior mandibular border for augmentation of vertical height, implant placement involves wide mucosal incision and subperiosteal exposure significantly beyond the dissection required for reduction of gonial angles in facial feminization including elevation of the pterygomasseteric sling. In cases where both gonial angle and chin implants are used for complete mandibular augmentation, extensive incision and exposure is required, possibly opening the entire length of mucosa from molar to molar. Implants

are seated based on specific anatomy of the buccal surface of the mandibular angle and ensured to be snug against the bone without soft tissue interference (see **Fig. 4**). The implants are then secured with 8–10 mm screws, the wound irrigated with antibiotic solution, and a watertight, running-locking mucosal closure performed with chromic suture.

Chin augmentation
Chin augmentation can be performed using alloplastic silicone or porous polyethylene implants

Fig. 10. Augmentation techniques for forehead (FMS).

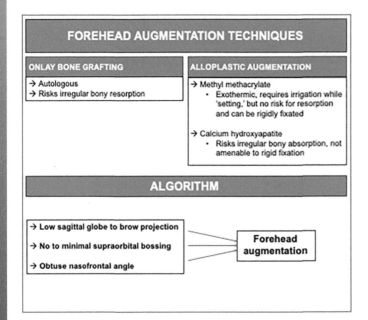

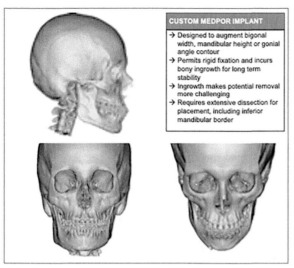

CUSTOM MEDPOR IMPLANT
→ Designed to augment bigonal width, mandibular height or gonial angle contour
→ Permits rigid fixation and incurs bony ingrowth for long term stability
→ Ingrowth makes potential removal more challenging
→ Requires extensive dissection for placement, including inferior mandibular border

AUGMENTATION TECHNIQUES	
TECHNIQUE	**NOTES**
Silicone Implant	• No rigid fixation, more easily removed
Cranial bone graft	• Can be placed between mandibular cortices via sagittal split osteotomy or in the belly of masseter • Does not require fixation • Invasive, risks resorption
Fat augmentation	• Augmentation of gonial angle/jawline • Can increase bigonial width but not mandibular height

Fig. 11. Custom implant/augmentation techniques for mandible (FMS).

as well as osseus genioplasty. As silicone implants are retained by periosteal attachments along the inferior aspect of the anterior mandibular border, they lack the ability to increase chin height. As a result, patients with deficient chin height mandated chin augmentation with osseus genioplasty. However, more recently developed custom porous polyethylene implants can be fixated to and extend inferior to the inferior mandibular border and offer another option for increasing chin height as well as projection.

Chin implants

We prefer custom porous polyethylene implants placed via intraoral gingivolabial sulcus incisions in the subperiosteal plane. Implants (see **Fig. 13**) are designed to extend distal to the mental foramen as they taper to meet the contour of the mandibular body without a discrete step-off. As a result, careful protection of the mental nerves is required during the extended dissection necessitated by the width of these implants. The implants are secured with 8–10 mm screws and the

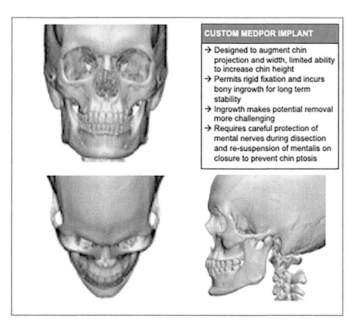

CUSTOM MEDPOR IMPLANT
→ Designed to augment chin projection and width, limited ability to increase chin height
→ Permits rigid fixation and incurs bony ingrowth for long term stability
→ Ingrowth makes potential removal more challenging
→ Requires careful protection of mental nerves during dissection and re-suspension of mentalis on closure to prevent chin ptosis

Fig. 12. Custom implant/augmentation techniques for chin (FMS).

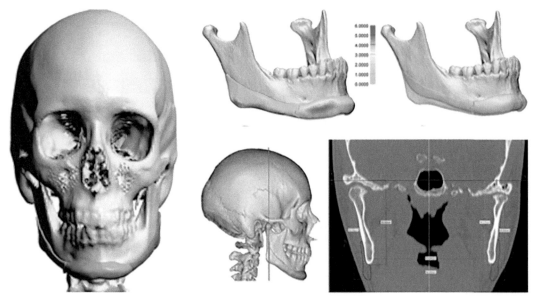

Fig. 13. 'Composite' custom implant for mandible and chin augmentation (FMS). Custom composite alloplastic mandibular and chin augmentation in facial masculinization surgery. Custom porous polyethylene implants can be designed for composite alloplastic mandibular and chin augmentation for increased bigonial width, increased gonial angle definition, chin projection, and chin width. Although typically fashioned in three inter-locking segments, such porous polyethylene implants still require extensive mucosal and periosteal exposure, sometimes necessitating complete mucosal incision of the mandibular gingivobuccal and gingivolabial sulcus. Careful identification and protection of mental nerves are required when placing composite implants. The coronal CT scan above demonstrates the planned dimensions of the custom implant, which fits to the specific anatomy of the buccal mandibular cortex and curvature of the inferior mandibular border. Full subperiosteal release of the pteryogmasseteric sling and inferior mandibular border are required to place the implants without soft tissue interference. (*Courtesy of* Justine C. Lee, MD, PhD, California, USA.)

mentalis resuspended. A water tight mucosal closure is then performed with running locking chromic sutures.

OUTCOMES/COMPLICATIONS

A small subset of studies have explored VSP and cutting guides within the realm of FFS.[14,19–21] A systematic review of all 3D and VSP technology use in FFS with or without intraoperative custom guide /plate use identified ten total studies that met inclusion criteria.[21] Despite limitations due to small sample size, absence of control groups, or few *in vivo* investigations, these studies have consistently unveiled enhancements in terms of safety, operational efficiency, and precision. For instance, Gray and colleagues's investigation showcased not only heightened precision but also reduced surgical duration, along with diminished instances of intradural violation and inferior alveolar nerve injury during FFS maneuvers in cadavers compared to a control group.[19] Precision was quantified by juxtaposing planned movements with postsimulation 3D CT reconstructions of cadavers. It is noteworthy that the utilization of guides exhibited optimal efficacy in forehead

procedures, whereas a somewhat reduced impact was observed in gonial angle ostectomy, primarily attributed to intricate visualization and limited access in this region.[19] Tawa and colleagues's study established VSP as a safe and accurate approach with robust patient satisfaction results, although their study design lacked a control group.[14]

Similar to prior work, our group has experienced no intraoperative or postoperative complications with our process of VSP and 3D cutting guides in a series of over 200 patients. Further, we believe VSP increases our operative efficiency as cutting guides enable facile osteotomies and preoperatively derived 'contour heat maps' from virtual mapping enable safe and expedient contouring of the calvarium without concern for causing full-thickness calvarial defects. Clearly, the need for comprehensive investigations persists to comprehensively gauge the extent of VSP's influence on operational efficiency and patient-reported outcomes within the landscape of FGAS.

SUMMARY

VSP enables high-fidelity transfer of preoperative surgical plans—carefully derived from clinical and radiographic assessment—to intraoperative maneuvers in gender affirming facial surgery. Key areas for virtual planning and cutting guides include forehead setback and recontouring, gonial angle reduction and chin reduction/genioplasty in FFS, and gonial angle and chin augmentation in FMS. Utilizing reference anatomic skulls for virtual planning offers a consistent approach to determine the extent of osseous maneuvers and allows for the simulation of various operative strategies. Custom guides and implants provide precise translation of surgical plan to the operating room by delineating the course of osteotomies, the depth of remaining osseous reduction, or specific anatomic fit of custom implants. Relevant studies demonstrate improved safety and efficiency with the use of VSP in FGAS; however, future investigations assessing the cost-benefit analysis and impact on patient-reported outcomes are required.

CLINICS CARE POINTS

- Key regions of the face manipulated with virtual surgical planning include the nasofrontal complex, superolateral orbit, mandible, and chin
- Preoperative clinical facial analysis coupled with patient-specific triggers of dysphoria is key for operative planning and postoperative patient satisfaction
  - Cephalometric analysis should also be performed and orthognathic discrepancies corrected before FGAS
- In FFS, osseous maneuvers are targeted toward bony reduction while in FMS, implants, augmentation, or genioplasty techniques target skeletal augmentation
- Use of 3D technology to compare patient and standardized anatomic reference skulls provides objective metrics for planning osseous movements
- VSP has been shown to decrease dural violation and nerve injury and improve operative efficiency. Future comparative cohort studies are needed to examine patient-reported outcomes in FGAS with and without VSP
- FFS specific pearls:
  - Management of the frontal sinus/nasofrontal complex is dictated by preoperative anatomy and can involve anterior table setback or burring. Custom cutting and contour guides demonstrate the depth of forehead reduction and outline the osteotomy for anterior table setback.

  - Osseous genioplasty with vertical and transverse ostectomies both narrow and shorten the chin. Rasping of the inferior mandibular border after advancement ensures a smooth contour without palpable step-off.
  - Gonial angle reduction with burring rather than ostectomy limits extensive periosteal denuding required to seat the large ostectomy guides and preserves the inferior aspect of the gonial/mandibular angle for optimal soft tissue draping and prevention of postop jowling

DISCLOSURES

The authors have no financial interests including products, devices, or drugs associated with this article. There are no commercial associations that might pose or create a conflict of interest with information presented in this article such as consultancies, stock ownership, or patent licensing. All sources of funds supporting the completion of this article are under the auspices of the University of California, Los Angeles, United States.

REFERENCES

1. Ousterhout DK. Feminization of the forehead: contour changing to improve female aesthetics. Plast Reconstr Surg 1987;79(5):701–13.
2. Ousterhout MD. Facial feminization surgery: a guide for the transgendered woman. United States: Addicus Books; 2012.
3. Deschamps-Braly, Jordan CMD. FACS Approach to Feminization Surgery and Facial Masculinization Surgery: Aesthetic Goals and Principles of Management. J Craniofac Surg 2019;30(5):1352–8.
4. Gilde JE, Shih CW, Kleinberger AJ. Frontal Sinus Transillumination in Cranioplasty for Facial Feminization Surgery. JAMA Facial Plast Surg 2019;21(6):566–7.
5. Cho SW, Jin HR. Feminization of the forehead in a transgender: frontal sinus reshaping combined with brow lift and hairline lowering. Aesthetic Plast Surg 2012;36(5):1207–10.
6. Altman K. Forehead reduction and orbital contouring in facial feminization surgery for transgender females. Br J Oral Maxillofac Surg 2018;56(3):192–7.
7. Altman K. Facial feminization surgery: current state of the art. Int J Oral Maxillofac Surg 2012;41(8):885–94.
8. Spiegel JH. Discussion: Osseous Transformation with Facial Feminization Surgery: Improved Anatomical Accuracy with Virtual Planning. Plast Reconstr Surg 2019;144(5):1169–70.
9. Spiegel JH. Gender affirming and aesthetic cranioplasty: what's new? Curr Opin Otolaryngol Head Neck Surg 2020;28(4):201–5.

10. Capitán L, Gutiérrez Santamaría J, Simon D, et al. Facial Gender Confirmation Surgery: A Protocol for Diagnosis, Surgical Planning, and Postoperative Management. Plast Reconstr Surg 2020;145(4): 818e–28e.

11. La Padula S, Hersant B, Chatel H, et al. One-step facial feminization surgery: The importance of a custom-made preoperative planning and patient satisfaction assessment. J Plast Reconstr Aesthetic Surg 2019;72(10):1694–9.

12. Kalmar CL, Xu W, Zimmerman CE, et al. Trends in Utilization of Virtual Surgical Planning in Pediatric Craniofacial Surgery. J Craniofac Surg 2020;31(7): 1900–5.

13. Chen Z, Mo S, Fan X, et al. A Meta-analysis and Systematic Review Comparing the Effectiveness of Traditional and Virtual Surgical Planning for Orthognathic Surgery: Based on Randomized Clinical Trials. J Oral Maxillofac Surg 2021;79(2):471.e1–19.

14. Tawa P, Brault N, Luca-Pozner V, et al. Three-Dimensional Custom-Made Surgical Guides in Facial Feminization Surgery: Prospective Study on Safety and Accuracy. Aesthetic Surg J 2021. https://doi.org/10.1093/asj/sjab032. sjab032.

15. Hoang H, Bertrand AA, Hu AC, et al. Simplifying Facial Feminization Surgery Using Virtual Modeling on the Female Skull. Plast Reconstr Surg Glob Open 2020;8(3):e2618.

16. Sayegh F, Ludwig DC, Ascha M, et al. Facial Masculinization Surgery and its Role in the Treatment of Gender Dysphoria. J Craniofac Surg 2019;30(5): 1339–46.

17. Morrison SD, Satterwhite T. Lower Jaw Recontouring in Facial Gender-Affirming Surgery. Facial Plastic Surgery Clinics of North America 2019;27(2): 233–42.

18. Dang BN, Hu AC, Bertrand AA, et al. Evaluation and treatment of facial feminization surgery: part I. forehead, orbits, eyebrows, eyes, and nose. Arch Plast Surg 2021;48(5):503–10.

19. Gray Rachel, Nguyen Khang, Lee Justine, et al. Osseous Transformation with Facial Feminization Surgery: Improved Anatomical Accuracy with Virtual Planning. Plast Reconstr Surg 2019;144(5):1159–68.

20. Mandelbaum M, Lakhiani C, Chao JW. A Novel Application of Virtual Surgical Planning to Facial Feminization Surgery. J Craniofac Surg 2019;30(5): 1347–8.

21. Escandón JM, Morrison CS, Langstein HN, et al. Applications of three-dimensional surgical planning in facial feminization surgery: A systematic review. J Plast Reconstr Aesthetic Surg 2022;75(7):e1–14.

Facial Feminization
Upper Third of the Face

Elie P. Ramly, MD[a,b], Coral Katave, BA[b], Kavitha Ranganathan, MD[a,b],*

KEYWORDS

- Facial feminization surgery • Gender-affirming care • Frontal sinus setback • Facial upper third
- Transgender care

KEY POINTS

- Facial feminization surgery (FFS) is a crucial intervention for transgender women.
- Key masculine and feminine anatomic differences characterize the upper third of the face.
- Patient-centered operative planning and execution ensure safety and efficacy in FFS.

INTRODUCTION

Facial feminization is a form of gender-affirming surgery designed to alter traditionally masculine appearing features of the face to more closely match one's gender identity. In the context of gender dysphoria, this is achieved through a set of medically necessary reconstructive procedures designed to comprehensively address the bony and soft tissue structures of the upper, middle, and lower thirds of the face.[1–3] For many transgender women, facial feminization surgery (FFS) is a critical surgical intervention that can facilitate integration into society. Recent advances in multidisciplinary care, preoperative patient selection and preparation, and virtual surgical planning have improved the safety and efficacy of these interventions.[4–7] FFS is associated with significant postoperative improvements in mental health related to depression, anxiety, and gender dysphoria and improves self-esteem, quality of life, and social functioning.[8–11] Unfortunately, coverage for FFS is variable across insurance companies and states.[12,13] Many patients still suffer from significant marginalization and limited access to experienced providers or centers where appropriate counseling, multidisciplinary care, and follow-up can be obtained.[12–14]

FFS can be performed in one or multiple stages and can be individualized to the patient's needs

and clinical presentation.[4,15–18] Gender-related esthetic standards are heavily influenced by racial, ethnic, generational, and cultural norms, adding a layer of nuance to FFS. In this article, we discuss reconstruction of the upper third of the face. Studies have demonstrated that our eyes are naturally drawn to the upper third of the face as a distinguishing factor in affirming one's gender.[19,20] As such, addressing the upper third of the face is one of the most powerful maneuvers in the gender-affirming surgeon's armamentarium for successful facial feminization.

ANATOMIC CONSIDERATIONS

Both bony and soft tissue structures distinguish the male and female upper third of the face.[20–22] Evaluating these structures systematically is critical in the process of preoperative planning.

The location of the hairline and shape of the forehead contribute to a masculine versus feminine appearance of the upper third of the face. The male forehead is longer, with a vertically oriented slope that increases in projection over the frontal sinus. The hairline is often receded in the temporal region, particularly in older individuals. In contrast, the female forehead has a rounder contour with a much less prominent glabellar ridge that transitions smoothly into the nasal dorsum without increased projection over the nasofrontal

[a] Harvard Medical School, Brigham and Women's Hospital; [b] Division of Plastic and Reconstructive Surgery, Brigham and Women's Hospital, Harvard Medical School
* Corresponding author. 45 Francis St, Boston, MA 02115.
E-mail address: kranganathan@bwh.harvard.edu

Oral Maxillofacial Surg Clin N Am 36 (2024) 183–194
https://doi.org/10.1016/j.coms.2024.01.002

region. The hairline is round without temporal recession, and begins approximately 5 to 6 cm from the glabella (**Figs. 1** and **2**).

The appearance of the abovementioned structures not only relies on modification of the soft tissue but also of the underlying bony skeleton. The frontal sinus is more prominent in men compared with women because of increased pneumatization during androgenic puberty. Altering the contour of the frontal sinus is critical to achieving a more feminized contour of the upper third of the face. Although classification systems exist to characterize the nature of the frontal sinus in detail, for the purposes of facial feminization, the main focus centers around the thickness of the anterior table. If the anterior table is thick enough, burring alone can achieve a feminized contour of the forehead. If, however, the anterior table of the sinus is too thin to achieve an appropriate contour with burring alone, as in 95% of patients, a frontal sinus setback is necessary. Preoperative imaging alongside thorough evaluation of the patient's photographs can guide the decision-making process.

In moving down the upper third of the face, masculine eyebrows are located at the level of the supraorbital ridge, and are much more horizontally oriented and thicker. Feminine brows are arched in shape over the lateral third, with the greatest

height located at the level of the lateral limbus of the iris. Feminine brows are located approximately 1 cm above the supraorbital rim providing a more open appearance to the periorbital area.

PREOPERATIVE CONSIDERATIONS

Proper patient selection is critical. We follow the World Professional Association for Transgender Health guidelines and obtain insurance authorization in preparation for FFS. A comprehensive history is collected. At our center, we allow patients to continue hormones perioperatively, and have a thorough discussion of risks and benefits. We require that patients stop smoking for at least 1 month before surgery. We do not routinely obtain laboratory studies unless patients have comorbid conditions or have a recent history of smoking.

Photographs and preoperative CT scans are performed to guide the decision-making process. We adopt a patient-centered approach by focusing on reconstruction of the areas that contribute most to dysphoria experienced by the individual patient. With regards to the upper face specifically, we focus on the patient's concerns regarding the hairline, upper and lower forehead contour, brow position, periorbital hooding, and nasofrontal region. We evaluate these features

A
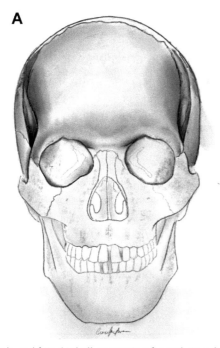

B
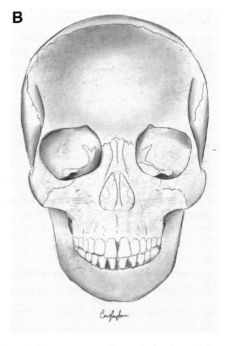

Fig. 1. Male and female skull anatomies: frontal view. (*A*) Male face anatomy: The male forehead is longer, with a vertically oriented slope that increases in projection over the frontal sinus. The male frontal sinus is extremely prominent compared with the female frontal sinus. (*B*). The female forehead has a rounder contour with a much less prominent glabellar ridge that transitions smoothly into the nasal dorsum without increased projection over the nasofrontal region. (*Courtesy of* Coral Katave, BA.)

A   B

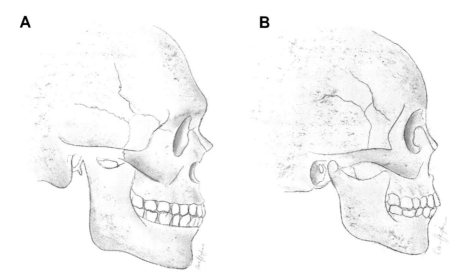

Fig. 2. Male and female skull anatomies: lateral view. (*A*) Male skull: lateral view. (*B*) Female skull: lateral view. (*Courtesy of* Coral Katave, BA.)

while also accounting for the structure of the middle and lower thirds of the face.

An important decision point regarding reconstruction of the upper third of the face is the choice of incision. To access the forehead and periorbital region, a coronal incision behind the hairline and a pretrichial incision along the hairline are both options. For patients with a round contour to the hairline, and glabella to hairline distance of 5 to 6 cm or less, a coronal incision is used. For patients with temporal recession, a receded hairline located greater than 5 to 6 cm from the glabella, or a masculine shape to the hairline, a pretrichial incision is recommended. Patients are counseled in advance that approximately 1 to 2 cm of hairline advancement is expected when the pretrichial incision is used. Such an incision can allow for excision of the temporal alopecia areas and advancement of the scalp and hairline, resulting in a shorter forehead and a more feminine-appearing hairline. The downside of this option is that the scar can be visible, particularly in patients who are prone to hypertrophic scarring or keloid formation, or those who prefer to wear their hair pulled back. Additionally, with age and changes to hormonal exposure or intake, the ongoing process of androgenic alopecia can eventually result in further recession of the hairline and an even more visible scar. This process can be slowed with medical therapy using minoxidil and finasteride (5-alpha reductase inhibitor), or counteracted with hair transplantation in well-selected patients.[23–25]

We use preoperative maxillofacial CT scans to execute the operation using virtual surgical planning (VSP) and computer-aided design and computer-aided manufacturing (CAD/CAM) technology to plan the bone cuts required for frontal sinus setback and orbital contouring. The frontal sinus cuts are made approximately 1 mm within the frontal sinus and follow the contour of the sinus closely. The orbital cuts are designed to resect the lateral prominence of the orbit that contributes to hooding in this region. Care is taken to make sure the cuts do not extend into the orbital roof or inferior aspect of the frontal sinus. We also design holes in the guide that allow us to maximize contouring of the entire frontal bone to maximize scalp advancement and feminize the forehead to the greatest degree possible. Burring to the base of these predrilled holes leaves at least 2 to 3 mm of frontal bone on completion, and maximizes uniformity of the burring process. Although FFS can be performed safely without these aids, we use this technology to improve operative efficiency and account for the individual patient's specific anatomy (**Fig. 3**).[5,23,24] This has also become a valuable teaching tool that can be used for preoperative and postoperative patient and trainee education and counseling.

PREPARATION AND PATIENT POSITIONING

The patient is placed in the supine position with the head at the top of the operating room table. The arms are tucked, and all pressure points are padded appropriately. A light shoulder roll is used. A foley catheter is placed. Although some of the smaller components of upper facial feminization could be performed in isolation under local or regional anesthesia, comprehensive upper facial feminization is

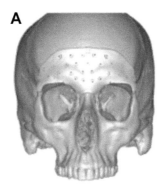 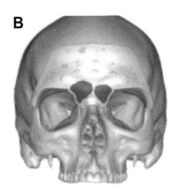 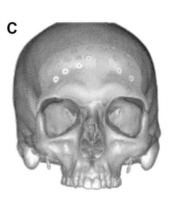

Fig. 3. Examples of frontal sinus guides accounting for nuances in patient anatomy. (*A*) Guide used for a patient with a thick frontal sinus. This guide facilitates uniform burring to achieve desired contour. (*B*). Guide used for a patient with 2 distinct frontal sinuses, which require separate osteotomies and set back. (*C*) Guide used for a patient with one large frontal sinus, which is osteotomized before set back.

performed under general anesthesia with oral endo-tracheal intubation. Depending on local operating room logistics and preferences, the bed is usually turned 180° to allow for a comfortable operating space. The eyes are protected with steri-strips. The incision is drawn in the pretrichial or coronal location, and a thin area of hair around the incision is shaved to optimize postoperative hygiene and surgeon comfort during closure. Local anesthesia is injected before prepping the patient. The entire head and neck is prepped into the field using beta-dine solution. Antibiotics are given preoperatively.

PROCEDURAL APPROACH

1. Incision is made using a beaver blade in a wavy pattern and with the blade beveled to optimize hair regrowth. The incision is carried through the skin and subcutaneous tissues to the level of the galea. Cautery is avoided as much as possible to prevent alopecia. Although the location of the incision is different, the same steps are used for the coronal and pretrichial incision types (**Fig. 4**).

2. Dissection is then carried straight down through the galea aponeurotica and through the periosteum to the bone using bovie electrocautery. A subperiosteal plane is created along the frontal bone between the temporal fusion lines.

3. Laterally, a knife is used to dissect down to the deep layer of the deep temporal fascia overlying the temporalis muscle. The soft tissues are undermined laterally at the level of the

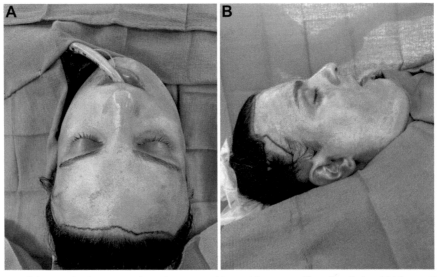

Fig. 4. Incision. (*A*) Pretrichial incision. The subsequent skin excision scar will end up being hidden at the hairline, allowing for brow lift and hairline advancement while shortening forehead length for a more feminine appearance. (*B*). Temporal extension of the pretrichial incision into the hair.

deep layer of the deep temporal fascia to avoid injury to the frontal branch of the facial nerve, which lies more superficially within the temporoparietal fascia. The subperiosteal plane and the deep layer of the deep temporal fascia are connected to form a uniform flap at the level of the temporal fusion line.

4. A periosteal elevator is used to dissect to the zygomaticofrontal suture laterally, below the orbital rims bilaterally, and approximately one-third of the depth into the orbital roof area (**Fig. 5**).

5. Care is taken to mobilize and preserve the supraorbital nerves bilaterally (**Fig. 6**). This happens naturally in the flow of the dissection in patients who have supraorbital notches instead of foramina. In patients with a supraorbital foramen, a 2-mm osteotome can be used to release the nerve to facilitate complete exposure of the supraorbital bar (**Fig. 7**).

6. Frontal sinus setback is indicated in patients with significant frontal bossing and a thin anterior table bone. The frontal sinus can be outlined using transillumination, and unroofed using a reciprocating saw.[4] Alternatively, preplanned patient-specific cutting guides can be used based on preoperative VSP and CAD/CAM. This is the senior author's preferred approach (**Fig. 8**).

7. The cutting guide is secured to the frontal bone using 6-mm screws.

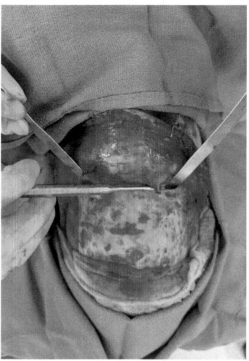

Fig. 6. Managing the supraorbital nerves (supraorbital foramen vs notch).

8. Because the cutting guide includes landmarks for bone reduction of the lateral orbital prominences, a piezoelectric saw and burr are used to remove bone from this area while being

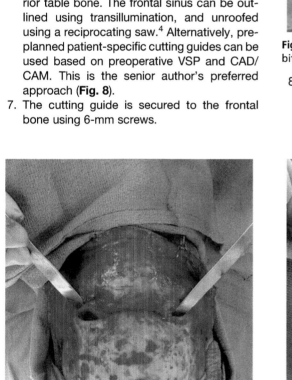

Fig. 5. Coronal exposure.

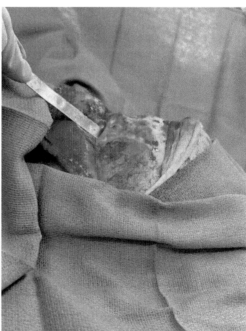

Fig. 7. Supraorbital dissection.

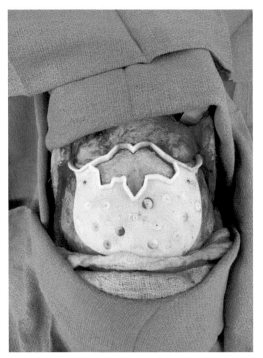

Fig. 8. Frontal sinus anterior osteotomy planning using three-dimensionally printed cutting guide produced through virtual surgical planning and CAD/CAM.

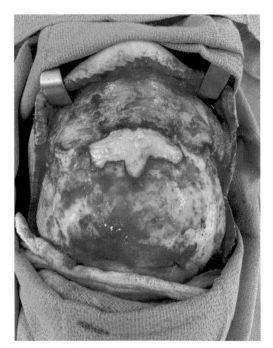

Fig. 9. Anterior table osteotomy.

11. The anterior table of the frontal sinus is contoured using a burr. It is then placed in a position appropriate to achieve the desired contour of the forehead while also optimizing

cautious to avoid extension into the orbital roof or communication with the frontal sinus. The frontal sinus is also cut using the piezoelectric saw. An osteotome is used to address any septations holding the anterior table in place (**Fig. 9**). The anterior table should come off in one piece with minimal injury to the mucosa of the frontal sinus and no injury to the posterior table or deeper structures (**Fig. 10**).

9. To optimize the extent of correction, we have small holes in the guide that are drilled using the 6-mm drill bit. The deepest extent of the hole indicates 2 mm of calvarium left in place for safety. Therefore, we are able to optimally reduce the contour of the forehead to facilitate scalp advancement while also optimizing safety throughout the procedure (**Fig. 11**).

10. The burr is used to reduce the prominence of the entire forehead and supraorbital rims. This feminizes the forehead and maximizes scalp advancement given the convex nature of the calvarium. This is performed until a smooth, curved, symmetric contour is obtained. We are careful to avoid burring on the inside edge of the frontal sinus because this reduces bone-to-bone contact, which can increase complications such as nonunion and bone resorption.

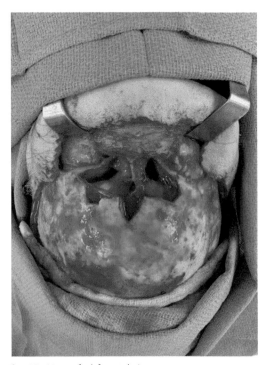

Fig. 10. Unroofed frontal sinus.

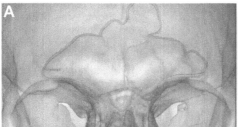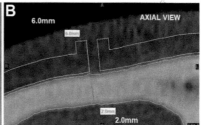

Fig. 11. Frontal sinus osteotomy cutting guide design. (*A*) The osteotomy begins approximately 1 mm within the frontal sinus and extends around the circumference of the sinus. This maximizes the ability to contour the frontal sinus and the surrounding frontal bone. (*B*) To ensure uniformity in the extent of burring, small holes are incorporated into the guide. These holes are drilled using a 6 mm drill bit. The base of the hole indicates that at least 2 mm of bone are present along the extent of the frontal bone.

bone-to-bone contact. Do not place the bone graft as an island because bone-to-bone contact is critical for a proper union. Two small plates are placed on either side of the frontal sinus. Four screws are placed in each plate (**Fig. 12**).

12. The tissues are irrigated and the bone dust collected during the process of burring is converted to a paste like consistency and used to smoothen the junction of the frontal sinus in its new position in a bone.

13. The brow lift is then performed by undermining the brows bilaterally and dividing the pericranium above at the level of the brows across the forehead. A 2-0 PDS suture is used to tack the lateral portion of the brow to the deep temporal fascia to feminize and elevate the brow.

14. The scalp advancement is performed by undermining the scalp in the subgaleal plane all the way to the occiput and advancing the scalp forward. A back-cut or excision of areas of temporal alopecia is designed to optimize hair-bearing tissue along the incision in cases where a pretrichial incision is used. The area of the forehead skin to be excised is marked after the tissues are appropriately tailor tacked

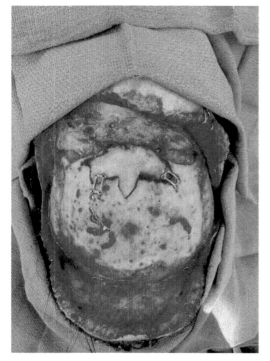

Fig. 12. Osteosynthesis of the frontal sinus anterior table after frontal sinus setback. If the anterior table fractures during or after contouring, it can be replated to restore its integrity.

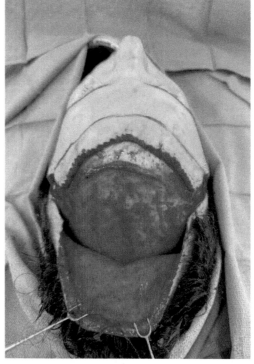

Fig. 13. Planning of frontal skin excision for brow lift before skin redraping.

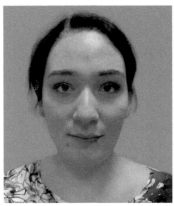
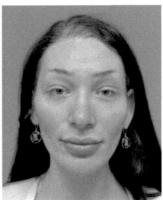

Fig. 14. Preoperative and postoperative frontal view. Patient is a 21-year-old transwoman who underwent hairline advancement through a pretrichial incision, frontal sinus setback, forehead/orbital cotouring, brow lift, septorhinoplasty, lip lift, and fat grafting.

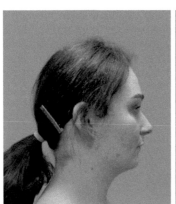
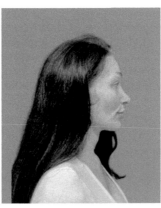

Fig. 15. Preoperative and postoperative lateral view.

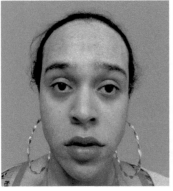
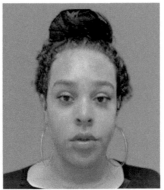

Fig. 16. Preoperative and postoperative frontal view. Patient is a 31-year-old transgender female who underwent hairline advancement through pretrichial incision, frontal sinus setback, forehead/orbital contouring, brow lift, lip lift, septorhinoplasty, and fat grafting.

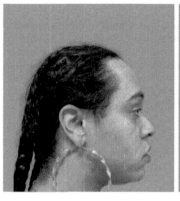 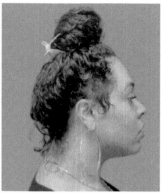

Fig. 17. Preoperative and postoperative lateral view.

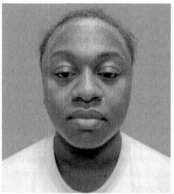 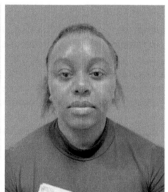

Fig. 18. Preoperative and postoperative frontal view. Patient is a 26 year-old transwoman who underwent coronal approach for frontal sinus setback, forehead/orbital contouring, septorhinoplasty, excision of buccal fat pads, and fat grafting.

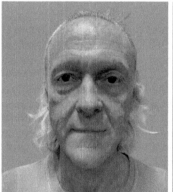 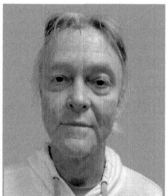

Fig. 19. Preoperative and postoperative frontal view. Patient is a 61 year-old transwoman who underwent hairline advancement through pretrichial incision, frontal sinus setback, forehead/orbital contouring, brow lift, septorhinoplasty, and fat grafting. Image shows results after second stage of facial feminization, which includes mandible reconstruction.

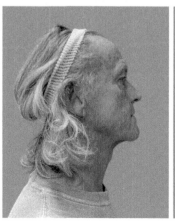 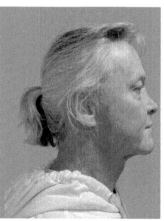

Fig. 20. Preoperative and postoperative lateral view.

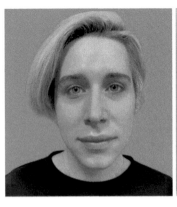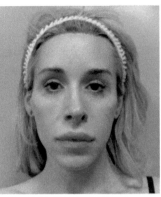

Fig. 21. Preoperative and postoperative frontal view. Patient is a 32-year-old transwoman who underwent pretrichial incision for hairline advancement frontal sinus setback, forehead/orbital contouring, brow lift, septorhinoplasty, fat grafting, and lip lift.

(Fig. 13). The marked forehead tissue is then excised, making sure that the brows remain symmetric.

15. To minimize tension on the incision, 0-Vicryl sutures can be used to advance the occipital scalp anteriorly. We do not perform galeal scoring for scalp advancement during FFS.

16. Layered closure is performed using buried 3-0 Monocryl suture placed in the deep dermis and galea followed by 3-0 Prolene sutures placed in a half-buried horizontal mattress fashion along the hairline. Horizontal mattress or simple interrupted sutures are used in the completely hair-bearing areas of the scalp temporally.

17. The tissues are thoroughly irrigated before closure and a 15 French round drain is placed in the plane of dissection and secured to the scalp.

18. Dressings consisting of Xeroform, bacitracin, and a headwrap using kerlix and an ace bandage are applied.

POSTPROCEDURE CARE

Patients undergoing upper facial feminization are typically observed overnight before discharge.

No antibiotics are used postoperatively. Patients can remove the headwrap after 48 hours and wash their hair. The subgaleal drain is removed during the first postoperative visit. Patients are counseled to sleep with their head elevated and apply Xeroform or Vaseline to the incisions with a head wrap as needed for the first week. After the first week, patients can switch to the ointment of their choice. We avoid prolonged use of bacitracin and other antibiotic ointments. Patients present for follow-up at 1 week, 3 weeks, 6 weeks, 6 months, and 1 year after surgery.

COMPLICATIONS

FFS is a reliable and generally safe operation in experienced hands but it is not without complications. Complication rates are reported to be approximately 1% to 5%.[26–28] The most common complications in our experience are wounds and temporary alopecia. Additional complications include hematoma, surgical site infection, chronic sinusitis, and hardware palpability.[27,29] Given the application of the anterior table as a bone graft, nonunion and malunion are possible but we have not seen this in our experience. Optimizing bone-to-bone contact is a critical aspect of

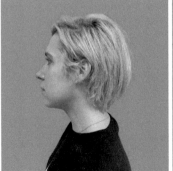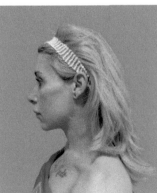

Fig. 22. Preoperative and postoperative lateral view.

preventing such complications. Using low-profile plates can reduce palpability of the underlying hardware. Because upper facial feminization involves extensive dissection and reshaping of the orbital rims, iatrogenic injury to the orbit and periorbital structures is possible. Stallworth and colleagues reported on 2 cases of superior oblique palsy after FFS, which resulted in persistent diplopia.[30] One case was treated with prism spectacles while the other eventually needed surgical management.

OUTCOMES

Similar to those of most facial reconstructive procedures, outcomes of FFS rely on a combination of subjective and objective parameters. With regards to objective outcomes, comparisons of before and after photographs, anthropometric and cephalometric measurements, and complication or reoperation rates remain the most commonly used and reported metrics (**Figs. 14–22**).[6,31,32] Although there is currently no widely accepted FFS-specific tool capturing patient-reported outcomes, there is literature to support the beneficial psychosocial impact of FFS, with reported postoperative improvement in anxiety, anger, depression, positive affect, meaning and purpose, global mental health, and social isolation.[8,9,33,34]

SUMMARY

Upper third FFS addresses anatomic features of the hairline, forehead, orbital rims, and eyebrows in order to induce gender-affirming changes that impart a more feminine appearance to the face. Proper patient selection, effective communication, and meticulous operative planning and execution are critical for success in FFS. The low-complication profile and efficacy of this operation in reducing misgendering allows transgender women to integrate more easily in society and highlights the life-changing impact plastic surgeons can have on this patient population.

CLINICS CARE POINTS

- For many transgender women, FFS is a critical surgical intervention that can facilitate integration into society.
- Upper third facial reconstruction is a critical component of FFS.
- Commonly performed procedures to reconstruct the upper third of the face include hairline advancement, frontal sinus set back, forehead/orbital contouring, and brow lift.
- FFS can be tailored to account for the individual patient's anatomy through thorough clinical examination and virtual surgical planning. It can be performed in one or multiple stages based on surgeon and patient preference and comfort.
- Coverage for FFS is variable across insurance companies and states. Many patients still suffer from significant marginalization and limited access to experienced providers or centers.
- FFS is a reliable and generally safe operation in experienced hands with relatively low complication rates.

DISCLOSURE

Nothing to disclose.

REFERENCES

1. Siotos C, Neira PM, Lau BD, et al. Origins of Gender Affirmation Surgery: The History of the First Gender Identity Clinic in the United States at Johns Hopkins. Ann Plast Surg 2019;83(2):132–6.
2. Spiegel JH. Facial Feminization Surgery/Gender Confirming Facial Surgery: Background and State of the Art. Facial Plast Surg Aesthet Med 2022; 24(S2):S17–9.
3. Spiegel JH. Facial Feminization for the Transgender Patient. J Craniofac Surg 2019;30(5):1399–402.
4. Eisemann BS, Wilson SC, Ramly EP, et al. Technical Pearls in Frontal and Periorbital Bone Contouring in Gender-Affirmation Surgery. Plast Reconstr Surg 2020;146(3):326e–9e.
5. Escandon JM, Morrison CS, Langstein HN, et al. Applications of three-dimensional surgical planning in facial feminization surgery: A systematic review. J Plast Reconstr Aesthet Surg 2022;75(7):e1–14.
6. Tirrell AR, Abu El Hawa AA, Bekeny JC, et al. Facial Feminization Surgery: A Systematic Review of Perioperative Surgical Planning and Outcomes. Plast Reconstr Surg Glob Open 2022;10(3):e4210.
7. Chaya BF, Berman ZP, Boczar D, et al. Current Trends in Facial Feminization Surgery: An Assessment of Safety and Style. J Craniofac Surg 2021; 32(7):2366–9.
8. Caprini RM, Oberoi MK, Dejam D, et al. Effect of Gender-affirming Facial Feminization Surgery on Psychosocial Outcomes. Ann Surg 2023;277(5): e1184–90.
9. Morrison SD, Capitan-Canadas F, Sanchez-Garcia A, et al. Prospective Quality-of-Life Outcomes after Facial Feminization Surgery: An International

Multicenter Study. Plast Reconstr Surg 2020;145(6): 1499–509.

10. Alper DP, Almeida MN, Hu KG, et al. Quantifying Facial Feminization Surgery's Impact: Focus on Patient Facial Satisfaction. Plast Reconstr Surg Glob Open 2023;11(11):e5366.

11. Chou DW, Bruss D, Tejani N, et al. Quality of Life Outcomes After Facial Feminization Surgery. Facial Plast Surg Aesthet Med 2022;24(S2):S44–6.

12. Aristizabal A, Escandon JM, Ciudad P, et al. The Limited Coverage of Facial Feminization Surgery in the United States: A Literature Review of Policy Constraints and Implications. J Clin Med 2023;12(16).

13. Hauc SC, Mateja KL, Long AS, et al. Limited Access to Facial Feminization Geographically Despite Nationwide Expansion of Other Gender-Affirming Surgeries. Plast Reconstr Surg Glob Open 2022; 10(9):e4521.

14. Ngaage LM, Xue S, Borrelli MR, et al. Gender-Affirming Health Insurance Reform in the United States. Ann Plast Surg 2021;87(2):119–22.

15. Telang PS. Facial Feminization Surgery: A Review of 220 Consecutive Patients. Indian J Plast Surg 2020; 53(2):244–53.

16. JU Berli, Loyo M. Gender-confirming Rhinoplasty. Facial Plast Surg Clin North Am 2019;27(2):251–60.

17. Hazkour N, Palacios J, Lu W, et al. Multiprocedural Facial Feminization Surgery: A Review of Complications in a Cohort of 31 Patients. J Craniofac Surg 2022;33(8):2502–6.

18. Siringo NV, Berman ZP, Boczar D, et al. Techniques and Trends of Facial Feminization Surgery: A Systematic Review and Representative Case Report. Ann Plast Surg 2022;88(6):704–11.

19. Spiegel JH. Facial determinants of female gender and feminizing forehead cranioplasty. Laryngoscope 2011;121(2):250–61.

20. Ousterhout DK. Feminization of the forehead: contour changing to improve female aesthetics. Plast Reconstr Surg 1987;79(5):701–13.

21. Schiwy-Bochat KH. The roughness of the supranasal region–a morphological sex trait. Forensic Sci Int 2001;117(1–2):7–13.

22. Bannister JJ, Juszczak H, Aponte JD, et al. Sex Differences in Adult Facial Three-Dimensional Morphology: Application to Gender-Affirming Facial Surgery. Facial Plast Surg Aesthet Med 2022; 24(S2):S24–30.

23. Tawa P, Brault N, Luca-Pozner V, et al. Three-Dimensional Custom-Made Surgical Guides in Facial Feminization Surgery: Prospective Study on Safety and Accuracy. Aesthet Surg J 2021; 41(11):NP1368–78.

24. La Padula S, Hersant B, Chatel H, et al. One-step facial feminization surgery: The importance of a custom-made preoperative planning and patient satisfaction assessment. J Plast Reconstr Aesthet Surg 2019;72(10):1694–9.

25. Capitan L, Simon D, Meyer T, et al. Facial Feminization Surgery: Simultaneous Hair Transplant during Forehead Reconstruction. Plast Reconstr Surg 2017;139(3):573–84.

26. Eggerstedt M, Hong YS, Wakefield CJ, et al. Setbacks in Forehead Feminization Cranioplasty: A Systematic Review of Complications and Patient-Reported Outcomes. Aesthetic Plast Surg 2020; 44(3):743–9.

27. Peleg O, Kleinman S, Ianculovici C, et al. Risk Factors for Postsurgical Infections in Facial Feminization Surgery. Aesthetic Plast Surg 2023;47(5):2130–5.

28. Chaya BF, Boczar D, Rodriguez Colon R, et al. Comparative Outcomes of Partial and Full Facial Feminization Surgery: A Retrospective Cohort Study. J Craniofac Surg 2021;32(7):2397–400.

29. Bonapace-Potvin M, Pepin M, Navals P, et al. Facial Gender-Affirming Surgery: Frontal Bossing Surgical Techniques, Outcomes and Safety. Aesthetic Plast Surg 2023;47(4):1353–61.

30. Stallworth JY, Hoffman WY, Vagefi MR, et al. Superior oblique palsy after facial feminization surgery. J AAPOS 2023;27(3):165–6.

31. Rochlin DH, Chaya BF, Rodriguez Colon R, et al. Secondary Surgery in Facial Feminization: Reasons and Recommendations. Ann Plast Surg 2022;89(6): 652–5.

32. Kurian K, Hao Y, Boczar D, et al. Systematic Review and Meta-analysis of Facial Anthropometric Variations Among Cisgender Females of Different Ethnicities: Implications for Feminizing Facial Gender Affirming Surgery. J Craniofac Surg 2023;34(3): 949–54.

33. Schmidt M, Ramelli E, Atlan M, et al. FACE-Q satisfaction following upper third facial gender-affirming surgery using custom bone-section guides. Int J Oral Maxillofac Surg 2023;52(6):696–702.

34. Alcon A, Badiee RK, Barnes LL, et al. Gender-Affirming Facial Feminization Surgery at a Public, Safety-Net Hospital: A Single-Center Early Experience. J Craniofac Surg 2023;34(3):1010–4.

Facial Feminization
Middle Third of the Face

Mona Ascha, MD, Bashar Hassan, MD, Fan Liang, MD*

KEYWORDS

- Facial feminization surgery • Maxillofacial surgery • Transgender • Rhinoplasty
- Malar augmentation

KEY POINTS

- Rhinoplasty and malar modifications can work in concert to feminize the midface.
- Goals of midfacial feminization are to create an appropriately proportioned nose, to achieve full and soft cheeks, and to attain midfacial ratios that contribute to feminine facial esthetics.
- The masculine malar region differs from the feminine malar region in both bony structure and soft tissue volume. Feminizing the malar complex requires addressing both.

INTRODUCTION/HISTORY/DEFINITIONS/ BACKGROUND

Facial feminization surgery (FFS) is a frequently requested surgical treatment among transgender and nonbinary (transgender and non-binary [TGNB]) patients assigned male at birth. Although planning for FFS is highly patient specific, common themes originate in addressing the upper, middle, and lower thirds of the face. For the middle third, attention is directed toward feminizing the nose and creating full and soft cheeks. In addition, interventions that address the sequelae of aging can also feminize the face, as soft tissue ptosis can obliterate the heart-shaped proportions of a feminine countenance. In doing so, attention must be paid to the transition between the upper and middle third. In particular, the periorbital to malar transition should be a smooth one, and the proper rejuvenation approach to the lower eyelid will complement changes to the midface.

As with other FFS procedures, modifications to the middle third can be incorporated within a single surgery or divided into stages. It is not uncommon for surgeons to address bony work along the craniofacial skeleton in the first stage (ie, frontal sinus setback, genioplasty, malar augmentation or zygomaplasty, and gonial angle reduction) and

soft tissue modifications in the second stage (ie, rhinoplasty, fat transfer, and rhytidectomy).

The goal with all the procedures is to optimize feminine facial harmony and improve gender dysphoria.

ANATOMY CONSIDERATIONS

The male craniofacial skeleton has distinct anthropometric characteristics that result in perceived masculinity. Ousterhout was the first to describe these differences as they relate to the TGNB patient, which include a prominent supraorbital ridge and frontal sinus, differences in zygomatic body proportions, and larger mandibular volumes.[1] Recent studies using geometric morphometrics and three-dimensional (3D) facial meshes have quantified facial sex differences for soft tissue as well.[2,3] In the midface, sex differences manifest in bony differences with the zygomatic width and prominence, the size of the piriform, as well as the size and thickness of the nasal bones. The soft tissue quality is sex specific as well, with men having thicker and more sebaceous skin, courser features around the orbit, and decreased fat deposition along the zygomatic prominence. As a result, the zygoma are less projected, with decreased soft tissue malar volume. The

Department of Plastic and Reconstructive Surgery, Center for Transgender and Gender Expansive Health, Johns Hopkins Hospital, 600 North Wolfe Street, Baltimore, MD 21287, USA
* Corresponding author. 600 North Wolfe Street, Carnegie 136, Baltimore, MD 21287.
E-mail address: fliang6@jh.edu

Oral Maxillofacial Surg Clin N Am 36 (2024) 195–205
https://doi.org/10.1016/j.coms.2024.01.003
1042-3699/24/© 2024 Elsevier Inc. All rights reserved.

masculine nose is more pronounced, with a higher nasal bridge, increased upper vault width, wider nostrils, a larger nasal tip, thicker sebaceous skin, and an underrotated tip.[2,4]

The cheeks and the nose are evaluated in tandem; full cheeks can detract from a larger nose, and a small nose can diminish the deflated appearance of flatter cheeks. However, by most accounts, achieving ideal malar esthetics in volume, contour, and position is best complimented by achieving feminizing rhinoplasty in the form of dorsal hump correction, nasal osteotomies, tip rotation, tip deprojection, tip cartilage refinement, and creation of a supratip break. One must however be wary of overcorrection; doing so can cause an uncanny valley appearance and draw unwanted attention to the aforementioned areas (**Fig. 1**).

Although most patients benefit from malar augmentation, one must evaluate the face in entirety. In some patients, the zygomatic width can be excessively wide, creating a larger and broader face, wherein the central features such as the eyes, nose, and mouth seem small. For such patients, zygomaplasty to reduce the lateral projection of the zygomatic body and arch may be incorporated into the operative plans for the middle third (**Fig. 2**). Within several cultures, large eyes and a small face are considered highly sought esthetic ideals.[5,6] When extended to FFS, interventions to reduce the overall size of the face, while augmenting the prominence of the eyes and lips, are feminizing. We see this perhaps most markedly in the aging patient, where soft tissue descent and accumulation of lower facial and neck adiposity increase the overall size of the face, particularly in the lower third. Ultimately, these

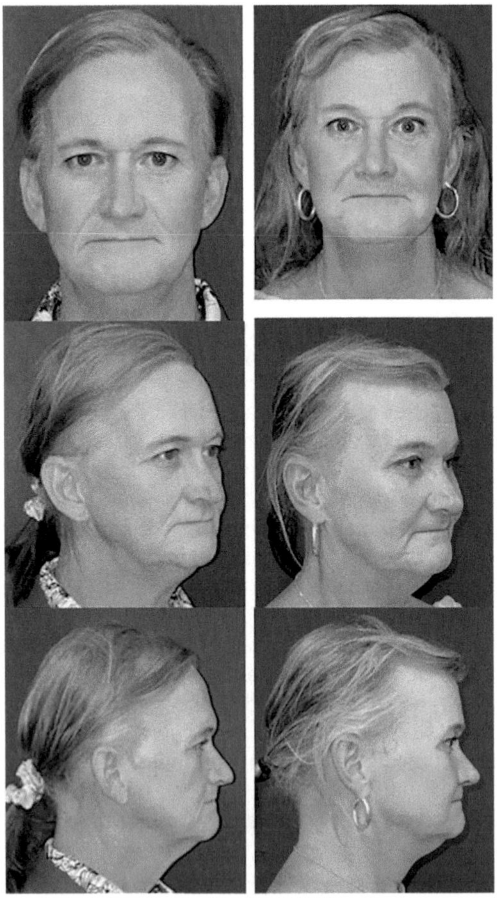

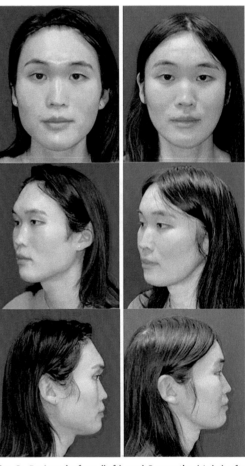

Fig. 1. Patient before (*left*) and 6 months (*right*) after single-stage FFS. Procedures included: frontal sinus setback, orbital rim contouring, brow lift, scalp advancement, facial fat grafting, malar PEEK implants, and septorhinoplasty.

Fig. 2. Patient before (*left*) and 8 months (*right*) after single-stage FFS. Procedures included: frontal sinus setback, scalp advancement, orbital rim contouring, brow lift, fat grafting to face, reduction malarplasty, gonial angle reduction, genioplasty, and tracheal shave. *Top row* shows the AP view, *middle row* shows the oblique view, and *bottom row* shows the lateral view.

changes transform even the most feminine faces toward androgyny over time.

GOALS/SURGICAL OPTIONS

The patient's surgical goals must be discussed and used to guide the surgical plan. The surgeon should set appropriate expectations for results and discuss what is achievable with each patient. On occasion, patients can present with both facial gender dysphoria and body dysmorphia; recognizing the latter is critical in setting attainable expectations.

Malar Augmentation

The male craniofacial skeleton often has a flatter zygoma, whereas increased anterior projection and softness is a sign of femininity and youth.[7] Toward this end, one must consider both the bony and soft tissue contributions to malar volume and shape. Malar implants correct the bony deficiency in zygomatic projection (**Fig. 3**). They give the appearance of having higher and fuller cheekbones and must be differentiated from the effects afforded by fat grafting alone. Implants neither change in size with weight fluctuations nor descend with age. However, malar implants pose an infectious risk and require revision surgery for explant. Implant-based cheek augmentation can be achieved with alloplastic malar implants made of silicone, porous polyethylene (PPE), or PolyEtherEtherKetone (PEEK). Each option has its advantages, as well as disadvantages. Silicone implants can be placed through smaller incisions, are customizable at the time of surgery, and can be easily removed.[8] They can migrate, however, especially if the pocket is overdissected at the time of placement. PPE implants are lauded in their ability to undergo tissue integration. However, they still can become infected and are difficult to remove once tissue integration is complete. PEEK implants are designed to register to a patient's individual anatomy, thereby making it easy to confirm proper positioning but are expensive.

In addition to implants, almost all patients seeking FFS benefit from malar and periorbital fat grafting. Patients without significant midfacial bony deficiency can be feminized with fat transfer alone. However, for most, the combination of fat grafting with malar implants is the optimal feminizing approach. Fat transfer accentuates soft tissue volume on top of malar implants and enhances the effect by increasing softness along the region.

Autologous fat grafting uses abdominal, superior gluteal, or inner thigh donor sites for transfer to the zygoma, periorbital region, temples, nasolabial

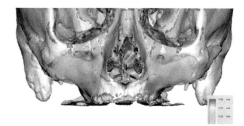
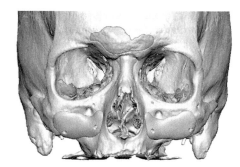
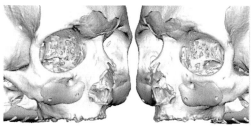

Bone Thickness Heat Map

Fig. 3. VSP of the above patient receiving patient-specific PEEK malar implants. *Top image* illustrates positioning of the implant relative to the malar bone thickness. *Middle image* illustrates optimal implant position between the zygomatic arch and piriform aperture. *Bottom image* illustrates an oblique view of implant placement, to visualize maximal bony malar projection. Note the extension of the implants to the lateral buttress to help with implant registration.

fold, and angles of the mouth. Some patients can benefit from fat transfer to the midforehead to accentuate the convex appearance of the feminine upper third.[9] Preoperative counseling should include mention of resorption of fat after transfer, need for serial fat grafting, and the fluctuation in fat volume with weight loss and weight gain.[10] This is particularly salient for the younger patient because body mass is anticipated to increase with each decade. The long-term consequences of facial fat grafting and the difficulty in removing excess facial fat have been documented by senior surgeons, who advocate for conservative transfer just above periosteum.[11]

Finally, malar augmentation can also be achieved during face-lifting procedures, with either plication of the superficial musculoaponeurotic system (SMAS) layer, or mobilization of the malar fat pad with deep plane techniques.

Reduction Malarplasty/Zygomaplasty

Zygoma repositioning and reduction, or reduction malarplasty, is a less commonly performed FFS procedure. However, it may be necessary in patients with pronounced facial width. This procedure has been popularized in Asian countries and among Asian women, who complain of excessive projection along the zygomatic arch (see **Fig. 2**).[12,13] The technique reduces facial width and creates a slimmer facial contour but must be balanced with the possibility of premature soft tissue ptosis as the facial skeletal volume is reduced. Excessive repositioning of the zygomatic body can also cause iatrogenic compression of the temporalis muscle and trismus. In the correct patient, however, zygomaplasty can be a powerful adjunct to midface feminization in patients with a broad and round face to achieve a feminine, heart-shaped facial contour.

Rhinoplasty

As the central component of the midface, the nose plays an important role in gender perception and attractiveness. The male nose tends to be larger, with wide nasal bones and a straight profile or dorsal hump. The nasofrontal angle in natal males is more acute, given the presence of a high radix, frontal sinus prominence, and dorsal hump. The nasolabial angle is also more acute, due to less nasal tip rotation and minimal to no supratip break. The male nose is also characterized by alar flaring and a more projected, underrotated tip. Feminization rhinoplasty is performed for nasal width reduction, dorsal hump reduction, refinement and rotation of the nasal tip, accentuation the supratip break, and reduction of alar width.[14] These maneuvers will also increase the nasofrontal and nasolabial angles to feminine values (see **Fig. 1**). It is important to consider functional goals as well as esthetic goals; both spreader grafts and inferior turbinate outfracture or reduction can be incorporated to ensure adequate airflow.

A nasal history and documentation of septal deviation should be recorded. Nasal skin quality, which may change with estrogen therapy, should be assessed.[15] Physical examination with a nasal speculum should document appearance of turbinates and septal deviation. Cottle's maneuver can be performed to assess the integrity of the internal nasal valve and the presence of alar rim grooving and alar collapse with deep inspiration can be used to determine the intrinsic support of the external nasal valve.

A key consideration in feminizing rhinoplasty is ethnicity and cultural context. Many patients may request a feminine nose but do not want overly westernized ideals. This should be part of the preoperative discussion and evaluation. It is recommended that patients bring in photographs of female family members and perceived ideals to understand patient goals.[15]

Buccal Fat Pad Removal

The buccal fat pad is encapsulated adipose tissue in the midface. It is located between the buccinator muscle and masseter muscle in the buccal space, and abuts critical structures such as the parotid duct, facial nerve, and facial vessels. The fat pad consists of a body and 3 lobes with buccal, pterygoid, and temporal extension. The buccal lobe contains about one-third of the buccal fat pad volume; the body and buccal lobe are the main parts of the fat pad targeted for removal.[16]

Appropriate patient selection for buccal fat removal is critical. Excess removal of the buccal fat pad or removal in thin patients with already hollow cheeks can lead to an appearance of premature facial aging.

Rhytidectomy

Rhytidectomy (facelift) procedures are usually performed in second-stage FFS after skeletal changes have been addressed. It is typically offered to older patients with evidence of generalized facial aging (>40 years). Patients should be evaluated for skin quality, skin laxity, dynamic and static rhytids, and facial fat distribution. Although several approaches have been described, the senior author prefers the deep plane approach because it affords the most robust repositioning of periorbital and midface structures, with natural appearing results. The feminizing facelift differs from its cis counterpart because the transmale skin and subcutaneous tissue is thicker and more vascularized, resulting in more intraoperative oozing when elevating the skin and SMAS flaps. The facelift is accompanied frequently with a necklift, with platysmaplasty and subplastysmal fat resection if necessary.

Masseter Muscle Excision

Cismales have a larger and hypertrophic masseter muscle compared with cisfemales.[17] Excision of a portion of the masseter muscle can achieve the desired feminine heart-shaped face. Surgical excision is sometimes preferable to neurotoxin injection because the latter requires repeat office visits and can become costly given the number of units required.

PREOPERATIVE/PREPROCEDURE PLANNING/ PATIENT EVALUATION

We recommend that surgeons adhere to the World Professional Association for Transgender Health Standards of Care v8 guidelines when evaluating patients for FFS.[18] Nearly all patients will be taking estrogen or antiandrogen therapy at the time of presentation. Although feminizing hormone replacement can be thrombogenic, the authors do not hold estrogen perioperatively. Instead, perioperative anticoagulation is administered, and patients are encouraged to ambulate immediately after surgery.

Gender-affirming hormone therapy can soften skin and slow androgenic hair loss; however, it cannot alter a masculine craniofacial skeleton.[19] With regards to the timing, it is imperative for patients to reach craniofacial skeletal maturity before undergoing therapy. This is typically achieved around the age of 17 to 18 years in individuals assigned male at birth, although there is variability in the age of maturation across different craniofacial areas.[20,21] Although a rhinoplasty may be performed at a younger age, significant manipulations to the craniofacial skeleton are not offered until the patient is aged 18 years or older.[22] There is no upper age limit for FFS, as long as comorbidities permit prolonged surgery and anesthesia time.

Standard clinical preoperative head and neck photographs are taken: frontal view, profile view, three-quarter view, and worm's eye view. At our center, 3D images using the Vectra imaging system (Canfield, Parsipanny, NJ, USA)[23] are also obtained for the assessment of soft tissue and to render the anticipated surgical result (**Fig. 4**). The authors routinely use thin cut (0.6 mm) computed tomography (CT) imaging for virtual surgical planning (VSP) of bony cuts for frontal sinus setback and genioplasty. In the midface, preoperative imaging is helpful for designing patient-specific malar implants that can be created that extend to the lateral buttress to help with registration at the time of implant placement. VSP for custom malar implants can be designed to maximize projection in areas of zygomatic deficiency, smooth the transition to the zygomatic arch, augment the bony projection along the piriform, and create inferior orbital rim support in patients with a negative vector (see **Fig. 3**; **Fig. 5**).

A systematic review of the use of VSP for FFS preoperative planning reports that VSP can improve operative efficiency, safety, and accuracy.[24] VSP can also improve safety because bony cuts are made within a safe distance of facial nerves.[25] However, its major shortcoming is its high cost.

A thorough medical history should be taken, with referral to any appropriate specialists necessitating surgical clearance. Just like many cis individuals, TGNB patients may have comorbid mood disorders, which should be optimized before surgery.[26] Perioperative counseling is recommended if patients have a therapist, and patients are warned about postoperative dysthymia. Preoperative laboratories, including serum cotinine (a nicotine metabolite), are obtained; surgery on active smokers should be avoided.[27] A focused facial history should be obtained, with particular attention to earlier facial or nasal trauma, prior facial injections such as botulinum toxin, filler, or silicone, seasonal allergies, and difficulty with nasal breathing.

PREP AND PATIENT POSITIONING

The authors routinely give a 1 g preoperative bolus of tranexamic acid (TXA) to reduce intraoperative bleeding. Although there is a concern that there may be increased risk of venous thromboembolism (VTE) among TGNB patients on estrogen, a retrospective study found no difference in VTE rates among TGNB patients undergoing FFS receiving TXA versus those who did not receive TXA.[28]

Patients are also given perioperative antibiotics, typically cefazolin.

PROCEDURAL APPROACH

- Malar augmentation
  - Bilateral gingivobuccal sulcus incisions are made after infiltration with local anesthetic.
  - The soft tissue and muscle are incised without skyving until the maxillary bone is encountered.
  - Dissection is performed in the subperiosteal plane over the zygoma and maxilla, with exposure of the zygomatic arch anterolaterally and piriform aperture medially. Care is taken to identify and protect the infraorbital nerve as it exist the infraorbital foramen.
  - Overdissection should be avoided because a large pocket can lead to implant mobility and malposition, particularly with the placement of silicone implants.[8] Adequate lateral dissection is necessary, however, to prevent dimpling along the skin at the lateral implant border.
  - The pocket is irrigated with povidone-iodine solution and/or triple antibiotic solution.
  - The implant is placed, evaluated, and fixated with 2 monocortical screws along the medial and lateral edge of the implant in the case of

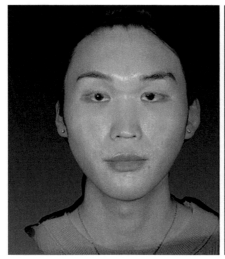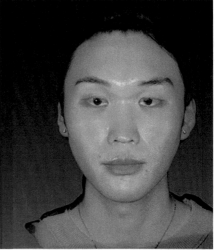

Fig. 4. Three-dimensional rendering of preoperative (*left*) and postoperative (*right*) results using Vectra camera. Note that only the midface was manipulated in the rendering (ie, upper and lower thirds of the face have not been changed). Facial narrowing of the midface region in the right photograph illustrates expected result from reduction malarplasty.

- PEEK and medpor implants. No fixation is necessary for silicone implants.
  - ○ The incision is closed in a watertight fashion with interrupted 3-0 Vicryl sutures along the mucosa.
- Fat grafting
  - ○ Fat grafting should be performed according to standard practices.
  - ○ A 4-mm cannula is used for power-assisted fat harvest, typically from the abdomen, flanks, superior gluteal region, and/or inner thighs.
  - ○ The authors prepare the fat using the REVOLVE fat processing system from Allergan Aesthetics (North Chicago, IL, USA).[29]
  - ○ Injection to the midface is performed with a 2-mm cannula in 1 cc aliquots using the Coleman technique of injecting into separate planes along the zygomatic body, periorbita, lateral orbital rim, temple, nasolabial

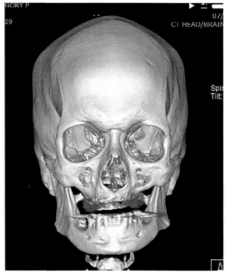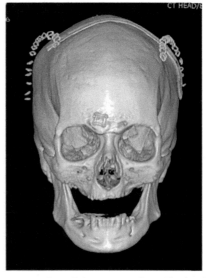

Fig. 5. Preoperative (*left*) and postoperative (*right*) CT 3D reconstruction of the same patient. The implants are in the appropriate position, several millimeters below the orbital rim, medial to the zygomatic arch, and lateral to the piriform aperture. They are safely secured with 2 monocortical screws.

fold, and inferiolaterally along the bilateral oral commissures.

- Rhinoplasty
  - Primary rhinoplasty is a complex procedure with many maneuvers; a detailed review of these maneuvers is beyond the scope of this article. Rather, focus will be placed on key maneuvers to feminize the nose.
  - The authors prefer an open rhinoplasty approach to achieve adequate exposure and surgical precision.
  - A transcolumellar stair step incision with intercartilaginous incisions are used to expose the lower lateral cartilages and nasal dorsum.
  - Transmasculine patients commonly require aggressive resection and burring of the dorsal hump; the authors prefer to use a reciprocating rasp for adequate resection. Excess septal cartilage is resected, and care is taken to resect the cartilaginous cap at the bony-cartilaginous junction to provide a smooth nasal dorsum.
  - Cephalic trim, leaving approximately 8 to 10 mm of cartilage, is performed to refine the nasal tip.
  - The septal cartilage can be harvested to correct any septal deviation and then used as a septal extension graft.
  - Autospreader grafts from turning in the upper lateral cartilages or traditional spreader grafts using harvested septal cartilage can be performed to prevent internal nasal valve collapse.
  - Low-to-low osteotomies with guarded osteotomes are used to obtain mobilization of the nasal bones; thereby narrowing the bony vault and improving the dorsal esthetic lines.[14]
  - Medial osteotomies to reduce nasal width can be performed if indicated.
  - Tip refinement is often necessary to feminize the nose, in the form of decreasing tip projection, increasing upward tip rotation, and decreasing tip width. The nasal tip cartilages are fixated to the septal extension graft and interdomal sutures are placed for the reduction of nasal tip width.
  - The authors prefer to use a septal extension graft for tip support and projection.[30]
  - If necessary, the alar bases should be addressed with wedge excisions. Additional techniques such as alar batten grafts, tip grafts, and crushed cartilage overlay along the dorsum are applied as needed.
  - Intranasal doyle splints as well as an external nasal splint are placed.
  - The incisions are closed with 6-0 interrupted Vicryl along the columella and 4-0 gut for the intercartilagenous incisions.
  - It is worth noting that if FFS of the forehead is being performed, the bony dorsum can be approached cranially. Radix reduction and grafting can be performed from this approach to achieve a gently curved obtuse nasofrontal angle.
- Buccal fat removal
  - There are several approaches for buccal fat removal; it can be combined with a deep plane facelift approach or performed intraorally. The authors typically perform the latter.
  - 0.5 cm bilateral gingivobuccal incisions are made, with care to stay away from the parotid duct of Stensen. Dissection is carried out along the lateral buttress of the zygoma.
  - External pressure is placed on the skin below the zygoma to herniate the buccal fat pad.[16] The protruded fat pad is clamped and excised with electrocautery. Only the fat that easily protrudes should be excised. Aggressive dissection and removal should be avoided to prevent hollowing of the midface.
  - Incision is closed with 3-0 Vicryl interrupted sutures.
- Reduction malarplasty/zygomaplasty (**Fig. 6**)
  - Bilateral gingivobuccal incisions are made to expose the body of the zygoma.
  - The anterior zygomatic body and anterior arch are exposed via subperiosteal dissection.[31] The infraorbital nerve is identified and protected.
  - A horizontal osteotomy below the infraorbital foramen is created, followed by 2 parallel oblique vertical osteotomies at the anterior portion of the zygoma, overlying the maxillary sinus. This creates an L-shape osteotomy and ostectomy.[31] The middle bone segment is removed.
  - Attention is turned to the zygomatic process of the temporal bone. A 1 cm incision is made along the anterior hairline/sideburn overlying the arch. A subperiosteal dissection is performed and an osteotomy is made with a reciprocating saw to complete the zygoma cuts just anterior to the articular tubercle.
  - The entire zygomatic complex is now free and can be mobilized more medially to reduce the width of the midface.[17,31] The zygomatic body is fixated with 0.8 mm plates and unicortical screws. Care must be taken not to overly medialize the zygoma along the arch because this can cause

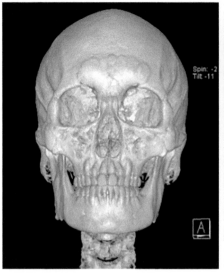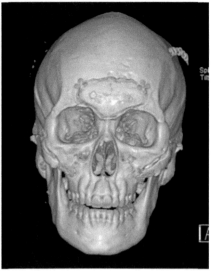

Fig. 6. Preoperative (*left*) and postoperative (*right*) CT 3D reconstruction of the same patient undergoing reduction malarplasty. Osteotomies were made along the anterior zygoma, with a portion of the zygoma removed. Osteotomies were performed along the zygomatic process of the temporal bone. The zygoma was then repositioned medially and plates were placed to secure the bony fragments.

impingement along the temporalis muscle tendon insertion onto the coronoid process and result in trismus.

○ The incision is closed in a watertight fashion with interrupted 3-0 Vicryl sutures along the mucosa intraorally. The anterior hairline incision is closed in layers with 6-0 Prolene for the skin.

- Masseter muscle excision
  ○ If a gonial angle reduction is simultaneously being performed, the masseter muscle can be accessed through the same incision. Otherwise, a 2-cm longitudinal mucoperiosteal incision is made over the external oblique segment of the mandible.
  ○ Subperiosteal dissection along the inferior and posterior border of the mandibular angle is made to elevate the masseter muscle off the mandible.
  ○ Reduction of the deep surface of the masseter muscle is performed, with excision of a portion of the muscle approximately one-third of its thickness. The muscle excised should be close to its insertion at the mandible border. If gonial angle reduction is simultaneously being performed, this is done before osteotomy.
  ○ Care is taken not to damage the masseter neurovascular bundle, which passes through the coronoid notch of the mandible and runs obliquely forward and diagonally downward across the deep surface of the masseter.

○ The incision is closed in a watertight fashion with interrupted 3-0 Vicryl sutures along the mucosa.

POSTOPERATIVE MANAGEMENT

We continue estrogen in the perioperative period because some studies suggest there is limited elevated risk of VTE among FFS patients on estrogen.[19,32] The authors do not routinely place head and neck drains, except after facelift/necklift. A head wrap and compressive dressing around the jaw are placed and worn for 1 week.

If the procedure has been extensive, patients are admitted overnight for observation and discharged on postoperative day one, as is standard practice.[33,34] Patients receive perioperative antibiotics, chlorhexidine mouthwash, and are placed on sinus precautions. Postoperative blood pressure management is critical in patients who have undergone face lift because hematoma is more common in cismales; clonidine should be prescribed for blood pressure control.

OUTCOMES

FFS is generally safe, with complication rates from retrospective studies ranging from 3.9% to 28.9%.[26,33,35–37] Most complications reported are minor, with the majority including wound healing issues and minor wound infection.

Although most studies on FFS report high patient satisfaction, few use validated patient-reported outcome measures (PROMs).[33] Further, among reports using PROMs, a wide variety of PROMs are used, indicating the need for a standardized FFS PROM.[38,39] This is currently being developed but has yet to be deployed on a large scale.[40]

One study reports approximately one-quarter of patients who underwent FFS requesting unplanned revision.[41] The most common reason FFS patients request unplanned revision is undercorrection of masculine features. The nose is the most frequently reoperated surgical site and the most frequent primary site of secondary surgery.[41]

NEW DEVELOPMENTS/FUTURE DIRECTIONS
Ethnic Considerations

Racial and ethnic considerations play a crucial role in FFS because they significantly influence the esthetic goals and surgical approaches. The distinct facial features inherent to different racial and ethnic groups necessitate a tailored approach to FFS. For instance, individuals from Asian backgrounds may seek adjustments to facial width through procedures such as zygomaplasty, which is less common in other ethnic groups.[12,13] Additionally, cultural perceptions of femininity vary, and this influences the desired outcomes of FFS. Surgeons must be cognizant of maintaining the ethnic integrity of the patient while achieving feminization. This requires a deep understanding of diverse facial structures and an appreciation of the cultural nuances that define gender expression within different ethnicities. Patients often desire a balance between attaining a feminine appearance and retaining their racial or ethnic identity, making a personalized approach and culturally sensitive counseling essential components of successful FFS.

Nonbinary Facial Surgery

Facial surgery for nonbinary individuals, similar to those undertaken by transgender individuals, focuses on aligning the individual's facial features with their gender identity, which may not necessarily conform to traditional male or female norms. These surgical procedures, often part of broader facial feminization or masculinization surgeries, are highly personalized. They aim to soften or accentuate certain craniofacial features based on the unique needs and esthetic goals of nonbinary individuals. Key areas of focus typically include the reshaping of the nose, cheeks, and jawline. The overarching goal of these surgeries is not just esthetic enhancement but also the alleviation of gender dysphoria, thereby improving the individual's quality of life and self-perception. In this context, the role of the surgeon is not only technical but also involves a deep understanding of the patient's identity and goals to ensure the outcomes align with their nonbinary identity.

Facial Masculinization

Facial masculinization surgery (FMS) for transmasculine individuals is analogous to FFS for transfeminine individuals but with inverse goals. FMS aims to enhance the masculine features of the face to align with the individual's gender identity. This involves procedures aimed at augmenting the upper, middle, and lower thirds of the face to achieve a more masculine appearance, considering both skeletal and soft tissue structures. Common procedures in FMS include frontal cranioplasty, masculinizing rhinoplasty, midface contouring, mandible augmentation, and thyroid cartilage augmentation.[42] Adjustments to the nose may also be performed to align with typical masculine esthetics, such as increasing the nasal bridge's prominence or adjusting the nose's width and tip. The overarching goal of FMS, similar to FFS, is to create a facial appearance that is congruent with the individual's gender identity, thereby aiding in the alleviation of gender dysphoria and enhancing overall well-being.

SUMMARY

Middle third FFS involves tailored procedures focused on reshaping the nose, cheeks, and addressing age-related changes to maintain a feminine appearance. The anatomic considerations in FFS are centered on the distinct differences in the male craniofacial skeleton compared with that of the natal female. Overcorrection should be avoided to prevent unnatural outcomes. Overall, midfacial FFS requires careful planning and understanding of both skeletal and soft tissue variations to achieve desired esthetic and functional results.

CLINICS CARE POINTS

Pearls

- Individualized approach: Every patient's facial structure is unique. Tailoring the surgical plan to individual anatomic differences is crucial for optimal outcomes.
- Comprehensive evaluation: A thorough preoperative assessment including 3D imaging and psychological evaluation can help in planning and setting realistic expectations.

Pitfalls

- Overcorrection: Avoid overcorrection to prevent an unnatural appearance, which can draw unwanted attention.
- Infection risk with implants: Patients are counseled regarding the risk of infection with malar implants. The senior author has had success with PEEK implants and has treated infection with antibiotics to good effect.
- Mental health considerations: Recognize the potential presence of body dysmorphia alongside gender dysphoria. Unrealistic expectations can lead to dissatisfaction postsurgery.
- Weight fluctuations and fat grafting: Educate patients about the potential changes in fat graft volume with weight fluctuations, especially in younger patients.

DISCLOSURE

The authors have nothing to disclose.

REFERENCES

1. Ousterhout DK. Feminization of the forehead: contour changing to improve female aesthetics. Plast Reconstr Surg 1987;79(5):701–13.
2. Bannister JJ, Juszczak H, Aponte JD, et al. Sex differences in adult facial three-dimensional morphology: application to gender-affirming facial surgery. Facial Plast Surg Aesthet Med 2022;24(S2):S24–30.
3. Toneva D, Nikolova S, Tasheva-Terzieva E, et al. A geometric morphometric study on sexual dimorphism in viscerocranium. Biology 2022;11(9):1333.
4. Gulati A, Knott PD, Seth R. Sex-related characteristics of the face. Otolaryngol Clin North Am 2022 Aug;55(4):775–83.
5. Chen T, Lian K, Lorenzana D, Shahzad N, Wong R. Occidentalisation of Beauty Standards: Eurocentrism in Asia. 2020. Doi:10.5281/zenodo.4325856.
6. Cellerino A. Psychobiology of facial attractiveness. J Endocrinol Invest 2003;26(3 Suppl):45–8.
7. Stowell JT, Jha P, Martinez-Jorge J, et al. Neuroradiology in transgender care: facial feminization, laryngeal surgery, and beyond. Radiographics 2022;42(1):233–49.
8. Weinstein B, Alba B, Dorafshar A, et al. Gender facial affirmation surgery: cheek augmentation. Facial Plast Surg Clin North Am 2023;31(3):393–7.
9. Schultz KP, Raghuram A, Davis MJ, et al. Fat grafting for facial rejuvenation. Semin Plast Surg 2020 Feb;34(1):30–7.
10. Vasavada A, Raggio BS. Autologous fat grafting for facial rejuvenation. In: StatPearls Internet. Treasure Island (FL): StatPearls Publishing; 2023. Available at: https://www.ncbi.nlm.nih.gov/books/NBK557860/.
11. Lambros V. Fat injection for the aging midface. Operat Tech Plast Reconstr Surg 1998;5(2):129–37.
12. Kim YH, Cho BC, Lo LJ. Facial contouring surgery for asians. Semin Plast Surg 2009;23(1):22–31.
13. Hwang CH, Lee MC. Reduction malarplasty using a zygomatic arch-lifting technique. J Plast Reconstr Aesthetic Surg 2016;69(6):809–18.
14. Flaherty AJ, Stone AM, Teixeira JC, et al. Feminization rhinoplasty. Facial Plast Surg Clin North Am 2023;31(3):407–17.
15. Berli JU, Loyo M. Gender-confirming rhinoplasty. Facial Plast Surg Clin North Am 2019;27(2):251–60.
16. Swonke ML, Sturm A. Feminization of the midface: cheek augmentation and buccal fat pad removal. Oper Tech Otolaryngol 2023;34:50–6.
17. Dang BN, Hu AC, Bertrand AA, et al. Evaluation and treatment of facial feminization surgery: part II. lips, midface, mandible, chin, and laryngeal prominence. Arch Plast Surg 2022;49(1):5–11.
18. Coleman E, Radix AE, Bouman WP, et al. Standards of care for the health of transgender and gender diverse people, version 8. Int J Transgend Health 2022;23(sup1):S1–259.
19. Haben CM. Gender-affirming hormone therapy: what the head and neck surgeon should know. Otolaryngol Clin North Am 2022;55(4):715–26.
20. Albert AM, Payne AL, Brady SM, et al. Craniofacial changes in children-birth to late adolescence. ARC J Forensic Sci 2019;4(1):1–19.
21. Costello BJ, Rivera RD, Shand J, et al. Growth and development considerations for craniomaxillofacial surgery. Oral Maxillofac Surg Clin North Am 2012; 24(3):377–96.
22. Deschamps-Braly JC. Approach to feminization surgery and facial masculinization surgery: aesthetic goals and principles of management. J Craniofac Surg 2019;30(5):1352–8.
23. Canfield Scientific. Vectra H2 3D Imaging System. Accessed December 28, 2023. Available at: https://www.canfieldsci.com/imaging-systems/vectra-h2-3d-imaging-system/?gclid=Cj0KCQjwqs6lBhCxARIsAG8YcDjQek9LaY90L5PXRW5QKhbAtJPayHiVXlbKr2Pfpo2COR0juiltQQ4aAgcoEALw_wcB.
24. Escandón JM, Morrison CS, Langstein HN, et al. Applications of three-dimensional surgical planning in facial feminization surgery: a systematic review. J Plast Reconstr Aesthetic Surg 2022;75(7):e1–14.
25. Kuruoglu D, Yan M, Bustos SS, et al. Point of care virtual surgical planning and 3D printing in facial gender confirmation surgery: a narrative review. Ann Transl Med 2021;9(7):614.
26. Chou DW, Tejani N, Kleinberger A, et al. Initial facial feminization surgery experience in a multicenter integrated health care system. Otolaryngol Head Neck Surg 2020;163(4):737–42.

27. Horton JB, Reece EM, Broughton G 2nd, et al. Patient safety in the office-based setting. Plast Reconstr Surg 2006;117(4):61e–80e.

28. Alper DP, Almeida MN, Rivera JC, et al. Tranexamic acid in facial feminization surgery: quantifying a high-risk setting with exogenous estrogen supplementation. J Craniofac Surg 2023;34(5):1452–5.

29. REVOLVE™ Advanced Adipose System. Accessed December 28, 2023. Available at: https://www.revolvefattransfer.com/.

30. Rohrich RJ, Durand PD, Dayan E. Changing role of septal extension versus columellar grafts in modern rhinoplasty. Plast Reconstr Surg 2020;145(5):927e–31e. https://doi.org/10.1097/PRS.0000000000006730.

31. Ma YQ, Zhu SS, Li JH, et al. Reduction malarplasty using an L-shaped osteotomy through intraoral and sideburns incisions. Aesthetic Plast Surg 2011;35(2):237–41.

32. Zucker R, Reisman T, Safer JD. Minimizing venous thromboembolism in feminizing hormone therapy: applying lessons from cisgender women and previous data. Endocr Pract 2021;27(6):621–5.

33. Tirrell AR, Abu El Hawa AA, Bekeny JC, et al. Facial feminization surgery: a systematic review of perioperative surgical planning and outcomes. Plast Reconstr Surg Glob Open 2022;10(3):e4210.

34. Salesky M, Zebolsky AL, Benjamin T, et al. Gender-affirming facial surgery: experiences and outcomes at an academic center. Facial Plast Surg Aesthet Med 2022;24(1):54–9.

35. Chaya BF, Berman ZP, Boczar D, et al. Current trends in facial feminization surgery: an assessment of safety and style. J Craniofac Surg 2021;32(7):2366–9.

36. Gupta N, Wulu J, Spiegel JH. Safety of combined facial plastic procedures affecting multiple planes in a single setting in facial feminization for transgender patients. Aesthetic Plast Surg 2019;43(4):993–9.

37. Chaya BF, Boczar D, Rodriguez Colon R, et al. Comparative outcomes of partial and full facial feminization surgery: a retrospective cohort study. J Craniofac Surg 2021;32(7):2397–400.

38. Morrison SD, Crowe CS, Wilson SC. Consistent quality of life outcome measures are needed for facial feminization surgery. J Craniofac Surg 2017;28(3):851–2.

39. Uhlman K, Gormley J, Churchill I, et al. Outcomes in facial feminization surgery: a systematic review. Facial Plast Surg Aesthet Med 2022. https://doi.org/10.1089/fpsam.2021.0293.

40. Morrison SD, Capitán-Cañadas F, Sánchez-García A, et al. Prospective quality-of-life outcomes after facial feminization surgery: an international multicenter study. Plast Reconstr Surg 2020;145(6):1499–509.

41. Rochlin DH, Chaya BF, Rodriguez Colon R, et al. Secondary surgery in facial feminization: reasons and recommendations. Ann Plast Surg 2022;89(6):652–5.

42. Patel NN, Gulati A, Knott PD, et al. Facial masculinization surgery. Oper Tech Otolaryngol 2023;34(1):69–73.

Gender-Affirming Facial Surgery
Lower Third of the Face

Phil Tolley, MD[a], Srinivas Susarla, DMD, MD, MPH[a,b],
Russell E. Ettinger, MD[a,b],*

KEYWORDS

- Gender affirming • Mandible contouring • Genioplasty • Chondrolaryngoplasty • Osteotomies
- Craniofacial surgery

KEY POINTS

- Facial analysis for gender-affirming procedures requires understanding of the sexual dimorphism that exists between masculine and feminine facial forms.
- Surgical planning within the lower face must account for the contributions of the soft tissue envelope and underlying skeletal framework, as well as the effects that aging has on these structures.
- Surgery altering the facial skeleton should be deferred until after the completion of skeletal growth to ensure stable long-term outcomes.
- Surgical techniques for feminization of the face are not exclusively reductive maneuvers.
- Appropriate feminization requires wholistic understanding of facial proportions and dimensions which are selectively adjusted to produce feminine facial qualities without creating iatrogenically unfavorable results.

INTRODUCTION

Central to all gender-affirming facial surgery and specifically facial feminization surgery (FFS) is the recognition of numerous anatomic differences that exist between the masculine and feminine facial form. Like many other species, humans exhibit a basic sexual dimorphism that includes phenotypic differences in facial structure and morphology. The driving force for the emergence of this sexual dimorphism is the differential effects of estrogen and testosterone on key end-organ tissues within the head and neck region. These hormonal effects enhance different features within the facial soft tissues and craniofacial skeleton to ultimately create the overarching appearance of a feminine or masculine face. Although some of these facial differences can be reversed or softened through exogenous hormone therapy, other features remain unchanged and require surgical correction to achieve the desired facial outcome.[1,2]

The characterization of facial sexual dimorphism in the context of gender-affirming surgical reconstruction is largely credited to Douglas Osterhout, MD, whose seminal work has laid the foundation for modern facial gender affirmation surgery.[3,4] Herein, he described how selective surgical alteration of the forehead, midface, lower face, and neck can be used to achieve a facial appearance that is congruent with a patient's gender identity. Although upper facial surgery is indicated in a greater proportion of patients, lower facial surgery remains an integral component of FFS procedures. Within the lower face, the lips, gonial angles, mandibular body, central chin, and neck all contribute significantly to the facial dimorphism that exists between feminine and masculine faces. The end-organ tissues of the lower face are responsive to

[a] Division of Plastic Surgery, Department of Surgery, University of Washington, Harborview Medical Center, 325 9th Avenue, Box 359796, Seattle, WA 98104, USA; [b] Division of Craniofacial and Plastic Surgery, Department of Surgery, Seattle Children's Hospital
* Corresponding author.
E-mail address: retting@uw.edu

Oral Maxillofacial Surg Clin N Am 36 (2024) 207–219
https://doi.org/10.1016/j.coms.2023.12.002
1042-3699/24/© 2024 Elsevier Inc. All rights reserved.

androgenic puberty and undergo changes which result in immutable masculine features which remain present despite the feminizing effects of exogenous estrogen therapy.[2]

ANATOMY

It is critical to understand the morphologic differences in the lower facial soft tissues and skeleton in a masculine face in comparison to a feminine face when planning for a feminization procedure. The perioral region of the lips, lower jaw, chin, and neck all demonstrate subtle yet critical differences gender morphology.[5] In a masculine face, the total upper lip height is greater and will demonstrate an increased ratio of cutaneous lip height relative to vermillion lip height further accentuating the appearance of a "longer" upper lip.[6] In the feminine lip, there is increased volume within the vermillion resulting in more equal height ratio between the cutaneous upper lip and vermilion lip.[7,8] Further enhancement of the vermillion to cutaneous lip ratio is why cosmetic lipstick is often applied to "hyper-feminize" the perioral region. Owing to an overall shorter upper lip height, feminine faces will ideally demonstrate increased dental display in repose (3–5 mm) when compared with masculine faces (1–2 mm).

In the lower jaw, the masculine mandible will exhibit increased gonial angle "flaring," wider bigonial divergence, taller mandibular body height, a tendency toward a flatter occlusal plane, bifidity of the parasymphyseal region, and midbody fullness along the continuation of external oblique ridge (**Fig. 1**, top row). Conversely, the feminine mandible will show more limited gonial angle flaring, narrower bigonial divergence, shorter mandibular body height, a steeper occlusal plane, a unified symphyseal region, and less prominence of the midbody continuation of the external ridge (see **Fig. 1**, bottom row).[9,10] These skeletal differences are further enhanced by contributions of the overlying soft tissues. In masculine faces, increased masseter muscle bulk imparts greater width and squareness to the lower face and enhances gonial angle flaring through increased muscle pull on the mandibular angle insertion sites. Increased soft tissue thickness in the central chin and mentalis muscle hypertrophy may further accentuate bony bifidity of symphysis imparting a soft tissue cleft, dimple, or boxy contour to the central chin.

In the neck, the thyroid cartilage's prominence is a stigmatically masculine feature. Before androgenic puberty, the male and female laryngeal frameworks are largely indistinguishable.[11,12] The thyroid cartilage within the larynx is end-organ responsive to the increase in circulating endogenous testosterone and undergoes rapid enlargement during the pubertal phase of development. This results in a doubling in anterior to posterior length of the thyroid cartilage and accentuating the superior notched prominence colloquially known as the "Adam's Apple."[11–15] This rapid sagittal enlargement of the thyroid cartilage is responsible for increased rates of voice instability and the ultimately deeper vocal tone seen in individuals undergoing androgenic puberty compared with those experiencing estrogenic puberty.[16–18]

Generalized facial aging also plays a critical role in lower facial anatomy and impacts both the craniofacial skeleton and the overlying soft tissues. Age-related facial soft tissue changes are characterized by decreased dermal thickness, loss of skin elasticity through collagen degradation, and volumetric loss in subcutaneous and deep fat compartments. There is inferior descent of the facial tissues due to progressive laxity in the retaining ligaments which separate the deep facial fat compartments resulting in visual segmentation of the facial subunits compared with the smooth transitions between these zones in the youthful face.[19–21] In the lower face, this results in the emergence of deep nasojugal grooves, perioral rhytids, mandibular jowling, an obtuse cervicomental angle and squaring of the lower facial contour. Skeletal changes are also implicated in the facial aging process. In the lower face, the mandibular body height, ramus height, and mandibular body length decrease significantly with age in both males and females, whereas bigonial width is preserved.[22] The volumetric bone loss in the body and ramus results in an increase in the gonial angle blunting the transition between the vertical and horizontal elements of the mandible resulting in a loss of jawline definition.[22] The loss of skeletal support exacerbates overlying soft tissue ptosis and increases the aged appearance of the face which has implications for facial feminization procedures which can involve selective skeletal reduction maneuvers in the lower face.

PREOPERATIVE ASSESSMENT

In 2022, The World Professional Association for Transgender Health published a comprehensive update to their evidence-based recommendations for the safe and effective medical and surgical care of transgender and gender diverse people known as the standards of care, version 8.[23] Herein, facial gender-affirming surgery was highlighted as one of the medically necessary gender-affirming surgical interventions. The inclusion of gender-affirming facial surgery was based on numerous studies

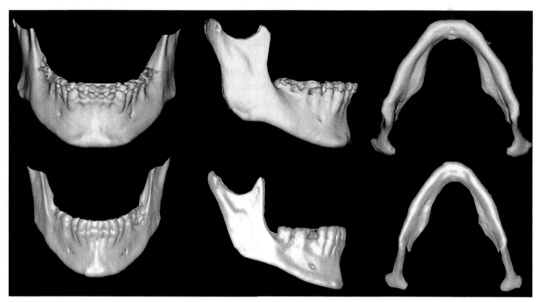

Fig. 1. Morphologic differences between a masculine mandible and a feminine mandible. *Top*: masculine mandible demonstrates wider gonial "flaring" wider bigonial divergence, taller mandibular body height, bifidity of the symphyseal region, and a square contour to the inferior border. *Bottom*: feminine mandible demonstrates limited gonial flaring, narrower bigonial divergence, shorter mandibular body height, and less prominence of the mid-mandibular body continuation of the external oblique ridge.

demonstrating that facial feminization can improve the feminine perception of the face, reduce misgendering, and significantly improve a patient's quality of life.[24–27]

Before surgical consultation for facial feminization patients will have met with both a primary care provider and mental health expert and obtained letters of medical readiness to proceed with gender-affirming facial surgery. These letters document that the individual has been thoroughly evaluated and deemed to be a candidate for surgery based on a current diagnosis of gender dysphoria and that all associated medical and mental health conditions have been optimized. The initiation of exogenous estrogen therapy for at least 6 to 9 months before consultation is advisable to achieve softening of the facial soft tissue envelope; however, this is not a prerequisite before surgery. The initial surgical consultation involves a completion of full history and physical examination. Details regarding an individual's social and medical transition can be sought to determine where they are in their journey and how different gender-affirming surgical interventions may help to achieve their goals of care. Exogenous estrogen therapy results in systemic effects which can be quite affirming (skin softening, decreased facial hair growth, fat redistribution, breast development, and decrease muscle bulk). However, there are often residual facial ques and features that can result in frequent misgendering

and exacerbate dysphoria. Asking which areas of the face create dysphoria for a patient is a reasonable way to initiate the discussion about different facial gender-affirming procedures. Prior surgical history, current mediations, allergies, and family history of disease should be documented. Special attention to prior facial surgeries including esthetic procedures and post-traumatic facial reconstruction should be elicited as well as prior use of permanent or temporary facial fillers and facial neurotoxin. A personal history or family history of venous thromboembolic events (VTEs) is especially germane to perioperative discussions for patients taking exogenous estrogen therapy who may have an elevated perioperative risk of VTE events.[28] A patient's smoking status and use of other nicotine-containing products should be evaluated as active use is associated with a significantly elevated risk of surgical complications.[29,30] Familial or social support systems should be elucidated as patients will require assistance with activities of daily living during their initial postoperative recovery.

Physical examination for the individual seeking gender-affirming facial surgery is done with a wholistic appraisal of the face with specific attention to the elements of the face which impart a stigmatically masculine facial form. Our typical approach is to have the individual sit facing the examining provider holding a mirror so that they can indicate the areas of their face which create dysphoria for them. Examination of the lower face consists of assessment of the soft tissues including skin texture and quality, cutaneous and vermillion lip proportions, upper and lower lip fullness, mimetic muscle thickness, masseter muscle bulk at rest and with volitional activation, and the presence of prominent submandibular glands. The degree of generalized facial aging is also assessed through evaluation of the skin quality, degree of soft tissue ptosis, and the presence of perioral rhytids, jowling, and nasojugal grooving. If there is a significant degree of generalized facial aging, then consideration for simultaneous skeletal advancement in addition to feminization should strongly be considered to avoid iatrogenic worsening of preexisting soft tissue ptosis.

Skeletal assessment is done via visual inspection combined with manual palpation to assess the morphology of the mandible including the degree of gonial splay, mandibular body prominence, bifidity of the symphyseal region, and vertical height of the mandible. Intraoral examination should note baseline occlusion, open bites, prematurities, degree of oral hygiene, soft tissue quality, as well as the presence of any masses or lesions. Examination of the neck should assess the cervicomental angle in profile as well as the visual prominence of the thyroid cartilage. Manual palpation of the thyroid cartilage can determine if there is a sharp cephalic notch or a broad sagittal prominence of the upper anterior cartilage which has implications for the degree of contouring that can be achieved during chondrolaryngoplasty without the risking destabilization of the vocal folds.

Standardized preoperative facial photographs are obtained as part of the initial assessment for patients seeking facial feminization procedures. The photographs are critical for documenting the baseline preoperative facial morphology and serve as a reference during subsequent virtual surgical planning. Facial photographs may also be required during the insurance prior authorization process to corroborate physical examination findings and support the ultimate surgical plan formulated by the treating surgeon. Once authorization for gender-affirming facial surgery has been obtained, a dedicated thin cut maxillofacial computed tomography (CT) scan extending from the vertex skull through the cervical spine is completed to evaluate the skeletal anatomy and cross-reference with the initial physical examination findings. Dedicated CT scan imaging allows for full characterization of the skeletal components of the head and neck and can be used for preoperative virtual surgical planning for computer-aided design simulations of bone recontouring and computer-aided manufacturing (CAM) of patient-specific cutting guides and fixation hardware (**Fig. 2**). The use of patient specific cutting guides and fixation methods can add material cost and surgical planning time but have been shown to decrease operative times and enhance surgical accuracy.[31] Standard facial bone series plain films consisting of an anterior-posterior, base view, and lateral views can be sought in lieu of a dedicated maxillofacial CT scan if virtual surgical planning is not being pursued.

When the decision to proceed to surgery has been made, the patient will return for a final preoperative appointment to review the surgical plan and make adjustments as indicated to meet the patient's goals of care. The antecedent risks, benefits, and alternative to FFS are reviewed with patient and include but are not limited to bleeding, pain, infection, wound-healing complications, sensory and motor nerve neuropraxia, dental injury, unfavorable scaring, hardware exposure/infection, osteomyelitis, and a need for future surgery. Urine cotinine screening to test for nicotine metabolites will be performed if there is any primary or second-hand smoke exposure. If the test returns positive, then the surgical case will be postponed to a time after which a negative screen can be completed. The elevated perioperative risk of active smoking and/or vaping in lower facial surgery is not inconsequential given that the vasoconstrictive effects of nicotine combined with heat generation can additively compromise healing of the perioral and intraoral incisions required to perform lower facial surgery. Patients taking exogenous estrogen therapy are advised to hold their estrogen for 3 weeks before surgery and 3 weeks following surgery to decrease their risk of VTEs. Although VTEs are rare occurrences, authors feel strongly that temporary cessation of estrogen therapy is warranted to avoid these potentially life-threatening complications. Individual surgeons should weigh each patient's individual risk of VTE in the context of age, preexisting medical factors, family history, and case complexity, and duration when determining their threshold for estrogen cessation for FFS until adequately powered studies can provide more robust evidence-based recommendations.

SURGICAL TECHNIQUES: LOWER FACIAL SURGERY

Sequencing of facial feminization procedures is at the discretion of the treating surgeon. Lower facial procedures may be performed in isolation or completed in combination with upper facial gender-affirming procedures. In our practice, upper face, midface, and lower facial surgeries are

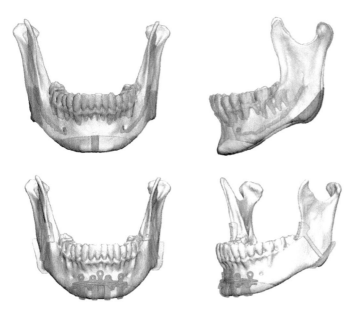

Fig. 2. Example images from presurgical virtual planning whereby computer-aided design (CAD) can allow for visualization of critical structures including tooth roots and the intraosseous course of the inferior alveolar nerve (*top*) and computer-aided manufacturing (CAM) can be used to generate patient-specific cutting guides and jigs to facilitate execution of the surgical plan.

carried out in a single-stage operation followed by inpatient admission for 24 hours postoperatively. Separating procedures can prolong treatment durations but can allow for surgeries to be conducted in an outpatient setting. Given the senior author's single-stage approach, orotracheal intubation with circumdental 24-gauge wire loop securement to a maxillary premolar is the preferred method of airway securement. This allows for access to the mandible around the endotracheal (ET) tube, which remains fully secured throughout the procedure. Flexion and extension positioning of the head and neck before definitive ET tube securement is confirmed by both the surgical and anesthesia team to ensure proper tube depth in all head orientations required for each stage of the surgical procedure. The ET tube is circumferentially covered with a clear, sterile ultrasound probe cover during final draping to further facilitate ET tube visualization and mobility during the case. Presurgical preparation for lower facial surgery includes placement of a throat pack followed by oral hygiene with chlorhexidine mouth wash. Presurgical IV antibiotic prophylaxis provides coverage for oral flora (ampicillin/sulbactam) and the face, head, and neck are prepped with antibiotic irrigation (vancomycin/gentamycin) given the need for concurrent full exposure of the entire head and neck region for multilevel facial gender-affirming procedures.

Lip Lift/Fat Grafting

The primary goal of a lip lift and autologous fat grafting is to increase the vermillion lip to cutaneous lip ratio. The former technique achieves

this through resection of cutaneous upper lip skin and shortening of the lip height, whereas the later achieves this through volumetric augmentation and unfurling of the red lip increasing lip height but increasing vermillion show. As such, careful analysis of upper lip proportions, lip height, alar base width, vertical maxillary height, and dental display is critical when selecting which procedure is most appropriate for each patient.

The superior incision line for a lip lift is marked along the basal contour of the nose at the junction with the upper lip skin. Lateral extension beyond the alar bases is not advisable as this creates a more conspicuous scar. Consequently, patients with a narrow alar base width may be suboptimal candidates for a lip lift as a primary feminizing upper lip procedure. The contour of the upper incision line can then be partitioned with vertical lines to facilitate accurate closure following skin excision. Manual manipulation of the lip can simulate the planned lip elevation and the lower extent of the skin resection is then marked conservatively to ensure eversion of the upper lip vermillion but without excessive exposure of oral mucosa beyond the wet dry junction. The resulting bullhorn configuration allows for effective elevation of the lip while providing a relatively hidden scar along a facial subunit boundary (**Fig. 3**).

With the area of upper skin resection delineated, local anesthetic with epinephrine is infiltrated to aid in hemostasis and the skin is incised sharply with a scalpel and dissection propagated down through the deep subcutaneous plane to the level of the orbicularis oris muscle with electrocautery on low settings. The skin and subcutaneous tissue

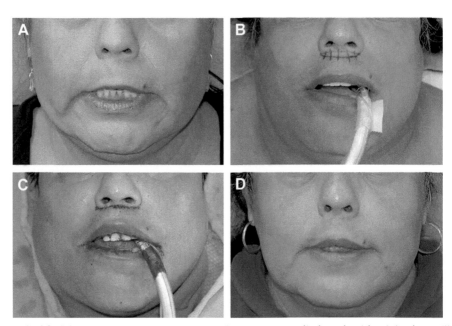

Fig. 3. Upper lip lift. (*A*) Preoperative appearance. Note long cutaneous lip length with minimal vermillion show. (*B*) Intraoperative markings of lip lift contained within the margins of the alar bases. (*C*) Meticulous closure following conservative cutaneous lip resection. (*D*) Final postoperative appearance at 1-year post-surgery demonstrating improvement in the cutaneous lip to vermilion lip ratio and a feminized perioral appearance.

is fully resected, and hemostasis assured with monopolar or bipolar cautery. Precise closure of the deep subcutaneous and dermal planes with meticulous alignment of the cutaneous landmarks is critical to minimize unfavorable scar healing. Closure is typically performed with 5 to 0 Vicryl in the subcutaneous and dermal planes followed by 5 to 0 fast absorbing plain gut and skin glue for final skin closure.

Autologous fat grafting to the upper lip is typically performed in conjunction with feminizing structural fat grafting to other areas of the face (malar regions, temporal regions). A central abdominal, lateral flank or superior gluteal donor sites are often used as these areas are readily accessible with the patient in a supine position. The selected autologous fat donor sites are infiltrated with a standard tumescent solution (0.03% lidocaine with epinephrine 1:1,000,000) and adequate time allowed for hemostatic affect. Given the relatively low volume of autologous fat needed to augment the facial region, hand liposuction is completed with harvesting cannulas on 30 cc lure lock syringes. Harvested fat is allowed partition from its heme and oil components which are then decanted. The fat is washed with saline and dried by hand rolling on telfa pads.[32,33] Fat can then be transferred to 1 cc syringes for aliquoting using the standard Coleman technique. Stab incisions at the lateral oral commissure allow for introduction of a blunt injection cannula into the substance of the upper lip at the level of the wet dry junction. A single passes with judicious injection of fat to optimize contact with adjacent tissue and avoid confluent tunnels is essential to maximize graft take. The volume of fat injected is titrated to individual patient needs but rarely exceeds 2 to 3 cc. Closure of the lateral oral commissure incisions is completed with 5 to 0 fast-absorbing plain gut suture.

Gonial Angle Reduction and Mandibular Contouring

The access to gonial angle region of the mandible is completed through a similar approach to performing an intraoral mandibular ramus osteotomy. A vertical incision in the mucosa overlying external oblique ridge and ascending coronoid process is marked extending from the maxillary occlusal plain superiorly to the first molar mesially. The location of the Stenson's duct opening should be visualized and marked to avoid inadvertent injury with incisional access. Mucosal incision is carried out after infiltration with local anesthetic with epinephrine submucosal dissection is carried directly down through the buccinator to the external oblique ridge and ascending coronoid region of the mandible. Periosteal incision is completed with monopolar cautery and subperiosteal dissection propagated to expose the inferior border, angle, and posterior ascending ramus of the mandible. A "J-stripper" can then be engaged along the inferior border and run distally and superiorly to fully release the pterygomasseteric sling off the mandibular angle. If mandibular body contouring is planned in addition to gonial angle reduction, the incision can be extended mesially to the level of the premolars. Our preference is to preserve intact mucosa overlying the mental nerve and limit the incisional burden but confluent access to the parasymphyseal region can be used if wide exposure of the mandible is required.

With the mandible exposed, several different contouring modalities can be applied to achieve the desired mandibular morphology. Mandibular ostectomies can be performed with the piezoelectric saw, reciprocating saw, or oscillating saw, whereas mandibular contouring and softening of ostectomy bone edges can be completed with high-speed rotary burs or power rasps.[34–37] Patient-specific cutting guides can be used to guide mandibular ostectomies which can be performed as true bicortical ostectomies or oblique monocortical ostectomies depending on a patient's anatomy and surgical goals (**Fig. 4**). Presurgical virtual planning can also aid in visualization of the intraosseous course inferior alveolar nerve in relation to the planned ostectomies and can simulate depth of burring to guide intraoperative decision making (see **Fig. 2**). On completion of mandibular contouring, the wounds are copiously irrigated to remove bone dust and hemostatic agents can be used as indicated. Watertight mucosal closure of the incisions is then completed with 3 to 0 or 4 to 0 Vicryl suture.

For patients with an angular lower jaw contour secondary to hypertrophic masseter muscles in addition to skeletal prominence, targeted chemodenervation of the masseter muscle can be performed with injection of botulinum toxin following mandibular contouring. The botulinum toxin can be delivered in three to four injections overlying the quadrangular region of masseteric insertion onto the gonial angle region of the mandible. Injections are kept inferior to a lone extending from the oral commissure to the ear lobule, above the inferior border of the mandible, and within the palpable margins of the masseter from anterior posterior. The authors generally use 30 to 50 U of botulinum toxin per side distributed across the injection sites but higher doses have been safely used for increasing effect.[38,39] Patients should be counseled that maximal muscle atrophy is typically seen at 2 to 3 months following injection.

Genioplasty

Incisional access to the parasymphyseal region is marked after noting the approximate location of the mental nerves in relation to the overlying dentition. The authors prefer an incision marked well above the lower buccal sulcus and higher on the lower lip to avoid foreshortening of the incisional cuff and to facilitate closure at the completion of the genioplasty. The mucosal incision is then completed and the underling orbicularis oris fibers are readily identified based on their transverse fiber orientation. Submucosal dissection is then propagated deep to the orbicularis fibers until the sagittal fibers of the mentalis muscle are identified. Once identified, the mentalis muscles are transected with monopolar cautery on low settings leaving a robust cuff attached to the mandible to allow for resuspension at the time of closure. Centrally, there is a natural diastasis of the mentalis muscle, so lateral identification can aid in ensuring an appropriate plane of dissection. With the mentalis muscle transected, the dissection plane is then brought directly down to the underlying symphyseal bone and a periosteal incision is made with monopolar cautery. Subperiosteal dissection is then extended mesially and anteriorly over the inferior border of the mandible. Distal dissection in a subperiosteal plan is then performed and the mental nerve can be safely visualized and isolated from an inferior to cephalad approach. Anterior fibers of the mental nerve may be encountered during the lateral extent of the superficial dissection and should be protected and preserved if possible.

With the soft tissue exposure complete the osseous genioplasty cuts can then be performed. The senior author's preference is to use preoperative virtual planning to guide the genioplasty cuts and final positioning of the bone segments through patient-specific cutting guides and custom plate fixation which allows for increased operative efficiency and precise positioning of the chin position (**Fig. 5**). Through the use of presurgical planning, level and angle of the genioplasty cut can be guided to ensure 5 mm of clearance from the inferior alveolar nerve course. Controlled, guided corticotomies are completed with the piezoelectric saw, followed by removal of the cutting guide and completion of the osteotomies with the sagittal saw. The specific maneuvers for gender-affirming genioplasty are highly patient-specific but generally require narrowing the width of the chin through central reduction which can then selectively be combined with vertical or sagittal lengthening to support the overlying soft tissue envelope. Central reduction in combination with sagittal setback and vertical height reduction should be used very selectively as aggressive reduction can result in destabilization of the lower facial tissues and create an iatrogenically aged

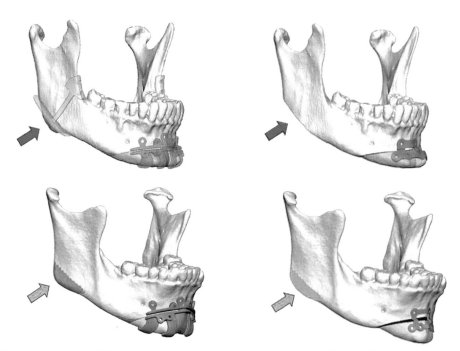

Fig. 4. *Top*: a true bicortical 90° gonial angle ostectomy (*red arrows*) guided by a patient-specific cutting guide referenced along the external oblique ridge. *Bottom*: oblique monocortical gonial angle ostectomy (*blue arrows*), simulated with computer-aided design to guide intraoperative free bone hand cuts.

appearance through soft tissue ptosis and the creation of jowling. Simultaneous sagittal and or vertical lengthening is not traditionally considered a feminizing maneuver but is powerful when done in combination with central narrowing to ensure filling of the soft tissue envelope and creating a refined chin point which contributes to the feminized "heart" or "almond" facial shape rather than the "rectangular" masculine facial form (**Fig. 6**). Irrespective of the genioplasty movements, the posterior segments are tipped up into posterior bony contact and any anterior bone gaps can be filled with interpositional bone grafts taken from the central chin reduction or from the ostectomies completed in the posterior mandible. Additional burring of the central segments and softening the transition to the mandibular body can be completed with a high-speed bur or power rasp as indicated.

Following completion of the bone recontouring and fixation the wound is irrigated with antibiotic irrigation and hemostasis assured. The mentalis muscle is resuspended to the preserved muscle cuffs to prevent a central chin soft tissue ptosis known as a "witch's chin" deformity and avoid lower lip incompetence. Watertight mucosal closure is a prerequisite given the presence of underlying fixation hardware with the propensity for oral secretions to dependently pool within the lower buccal sulcus.

Chondrolaryngoplasty

Multiple techniques for chondrolaryngoplasty have been developed since the procedure's inception but generally involve variations of either a direct transcutaneous approach or remote transoral approach.[40,41] Both methods are safe and effective but offer different advantages and disadvantages. The transcutaneous approach allows for direct exposure and visualization of the laryngeal cartilage but necessitates a visible scar on the anterior neck. Transoral approaches obviate the need for a visible cutaneous scar but require additional time, equipment, and advanced experience with endoscopic surgery. Our approach is done with a direct approach through a 2-cm incision placed superior the level of the thyroid cartilage at the confluence of the cervicomental junction or selected to coincide with a transverse neck rhytid (**Fig. 7**). Before initiating the exposure, the anesthetic oxygen concentration is decreased to at least 30% Fio_2 and minimal use of cautery is used to reduce the risk of airway fire. The skin is then infiltrated with local anesthetic with epinephrine. Following incision, subcutaneous dissection is propagated down to the level of the strap muscles with blunt surgical spreads through the midline raphe until the thyroid cartilage is identified. The pretracheal fascia is opened and the tracheal perichondrium incised with a scalpel.

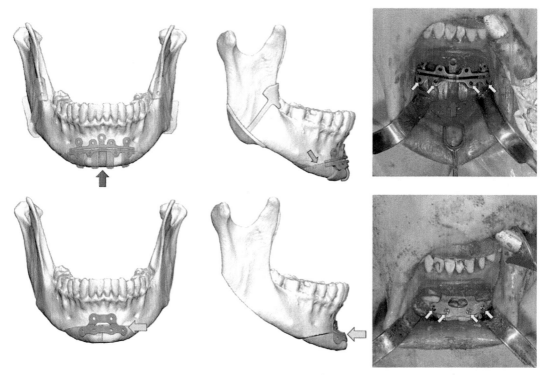

Fig. 5. Feminizing genioplasty aided by creation of patient-specific cutting guide and custom titanium fixation plate. *Top*: virtual surgical planning of a patient-specific cutting guide to perform 6 mm central narrowing of symphyseal region (*red arrow*) and a guided genioplasty cut with 5 mm of clearance from intraosseous course of inferior alveolar nerve (*blue arrow*). *Bottom*: final postoperative positioning of genioplasty segments controlled with patient-specific titanium fixation plate (*green arrow*) secured with predrilled holes from cutting guide (*yellow arrows*).

Subperichondrial exposure of the leading edge of the thyroid cartilage is then performed with a Woodson elevator exposing the anterior thyroid notch. With the cartilaginous prominence fully visualized, the anesthesia team will introduce a flexible bronchoscope through the mouth and visualize the anterior commissure of the vocal folds and the ET tube. Some surgeons and anesthetic teams prefer to use an laryngeal mask airway (LMA) in lieu of an ET to facilitate this visualization. A 27-gauge needle can then be introduced by the surgical team at the inferior most extent of the planned cartilaginous resection and the cephalad to caudad position of the needle can be verified to be above the level of the true vocal folds bronchscopically. This confirmation ensures that the planned cartilaginous resection does not extend below the level of the vocal fold insertion which would result in destabilization of the vocal cords resulting in iatrogenic deepening of the vocal tone. As such, some anatomic variations may not allow for complete flattening of the thyroid prominence without undue risk for vocal alteration which should be disclosed to patients preoperatively. With the inferior extent of the

cartilaginous resection marked, the bronchoscope and transcartilaginous needle can be removed. Contouring of the thyroid cartilage can then be iteratively completed with a diamond tip high-speed bur. Visualization and manual palpation confirm the desired result (see **Fig. 7**). The surgical site is then copiously irrigated with antibiotic irrigation and checked for inadvertent airway violation with a Valsalva maneuver with the operative site submerged with irrigation. Closure is layers of the pretracheal fascia, deep subcutaneous tissue, and dermis can then be performed with absorbable suture.

POSTOPERATIVE CARE

Gender-affirming lower jaw procedures can be completed within an outpatient setting but often are completed concurrently with upper facial gender-affirming surgery. Postoperative admission for 24 hours is typical for single-stage full facial feminization procedures to allow adequate time to achieve pain control and sufficient oral intake and hydration. Lower facial edema can be considerable following the multilevel facial

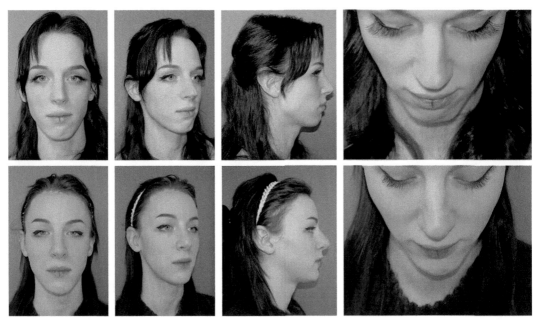

Fig. 6. Feminizing genioplasty via central narrowing, vertical lengthening, and sagittal advancement. *Top*: presurgical facial photographs demonstrating retrognathic chin position with boxy and angular contour of symphyseal region and evidence of mentalis strain to achieve oral competence signifying lack of skeletal support to overlying soft tissue envelope within the lower third of the face. *Bottom*: postoperative facial photographs 1 year following feminizing genioplasty via central narrowing, vertical lengthening, and sagittal advancement. Note morphologic feminization of the lower third through the creation of a single unifying chin, a "V" shaped inferior border contour, and filling of the overlying soft tissue envelope through skeletal expansion and the resultant resolution of mentalis strain.

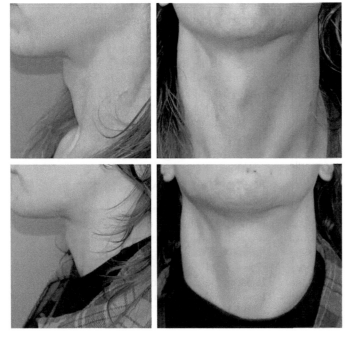

Fig. 7. Feminizing chondrolaryngoplasty via direct transcutaneous approach. *Top*: presurgical appearance with prominence of the thyroid cartilage. *Bottom*: postoperative appearance with reduction in the cephalic prominence of thyroid cartilage.

procedures which is further accentuated by the dependent gravitational collection of upper facial edema. Strict head of bed elevation and facial compression garments are mainstays of management. Ice may be used within the first 24 hours to further assist with edema control but should not be directly applied to the skin or excessive periods of time to avoid cold injury due to diminished peripheral sensation. Oral care with twice daily chlorhexidine mouth wash and saltwater rinses after meals is instituted with transition to over-the-counter mouth wash at 7 days postoperatively. Gentle tooth brushing with a soft bristle toothbrush is initiated at 48 hours postoperatively and a soft nonmasticatory diet is maintained for 3-week postoperatively or until the intraoral can be verified to be healing appropriately. Postoperative antibiotic prophylaxis is only maintained during the hospital stay. Facial compression therapy is strictly maintained for 6-week postoperatively to allow for readaptation of the soft tissue to the recontoured mandible profile. Patients are counseled that improvements in the lower facial profile may take several months to become visible due to slower recession of lower facial edema when compared with upper facial changes.

COMPLICATIONS

Complications of lower facial gender-affirming surgery parallel the expected complication profiles for other soft tissue and bony surgeries performed within the lower face. Complications range from more common postsurgical concerns such as bleeding, pain, infection, unfavorable scaring, sensory disturbance, and wound-healing complications to more rare or serious complications such as unfavorable osteotomy propagation, long-term contour asymmetries, hardware exposure, osteomyelitis, malunion, non-union, and hardware failures. Patients should be counseled on the full extent of the associated complications, but large series on facial feminization have demonstrated overall low rates complications many of which can be resolved with conservative or expectant management.[42–45]

SUMMARY

Lower facial surgery is a critical component within the compendium of gender-affirming facial surgery procedures. Lower facial procedures are specifically focused on addressing both the soft tissue and bony contributions to facial dimorphism that exists between a masculine and feminine face. A wholistic understanding of facial gender morphology and measured appraisal of

each individual patient's presenting concerns in relation to their baseline facial anatomy is essential to develop a treatment plan which achieves the desired outcomes. Selective skeletal reduction is often necessary to soften the angular qualities of a masculine face, but care should be exercised to avoid iatrogenic destabilization of the overlying soft tissues resulting in a prematurely aged appearance. The craniofacial principle of skeletal expansion to fill the overlying soft tissues is readily applicable within lower facial gender-affirming surgery and can synergize with concurrent upper facial surgery to achieve dramatic feminization of the face which can alleviate gender dysphoria, increase mental health, and improve quality of life.[26,27,46]

CLINICS CARE POINTS

- The lower face harbors key dimorphic differences that differentiate the masculine and feminine facial form.
- Incorporation of patient driven concerns regarding specific facial features that cause dysphoria are essential to the pre-surgical planning process.
- Individual appraisal of both the soft tissue and skeletal framework of the lower face is critical when evaluating a patient for feminizing lower facial surgery.
- Presurgical virtual planning is not a prerequisite but can be utilized to increase intraoperative safety and efficiency in lower facial procedures.
- Reliance on only reductive maneuvers in lower facial gender affirming surgery can result in iatrogenic soft tissue destabilization and a prematurely aged appearance.
- Selective advancement and lengthening, particularly within the bony skeleton, can provide a feminized appearance while simultaneously supporting the overlying soft tissue envelope.

DISCLOSURE

The authors have nothing to disclose.

REFERENCES

1. Hembree WC, Cohen-Kettenis PT, Gooren L, et al. Endocrine treatment of gender-dysphoric/gender-

incongruent persons: an endocrine society clinical practice guideline. Endocr Pract 2017;23(12):1437.

2. Marečková K, Weinbrand Z, Chakravarty MM, et al. Testosterone-mediated sex differences in the face shape during adolescence: subjective impressions and objective features. Horm Behav 2011;60(5):681–90.

3. Ousterhout DK. Feminization of the forehead: contour changing to improve female aesthetics. Plast Reconstr Surg 1987;79(5):701–13.

4. Ousterhout DK. Aesthetic contouring of the craniofacial skeleton. 1st edition. New York, NY: Little, Brown and Company; 1991.

5. Morrison SD, Satterwhite T. Lower Jaw Recontouring in Facial Gender-Affirming Surgery. Facial Plast Surg Clin North Am 2019;27(2):233–42.

6. Farkas LG, Katic MJ, Hreczko TA, et al. Anthropometric proportions in the upper lip-lower lip-chin area of the lower face in young white adults. Am J Orthod 1984;86(1):52–60.

7. Penna V, Fricke A, Iblher N, et al. The attractive lip: a photomorphometric analysis. J Plast Reconstr Aesthet Surg 2015;68(7):920–9.

8. Anic-Milosevic S, Mestrovic S, Prlić A, et al. Proportions in the upper lip-lower lip-chin area of the lower face as determined by photogrammetric method. J Cranio-Maxillo-Fac Surg 2010;38(2):90–5.

9. Thayer ZM, Dobson SD. Sexual dimorphism in chin shape: implications for adaptive hypotheses. Am J Phys Anthropol 2010;143(3):417–25.

10. Coquerelle M, Bookstein FL, Braga J, et al. Sexual dimorphism of the human mandible and its association with dental development. Am J Phys Anthropol 2011;145(2):192–202.

11. Kahane JC. A morphological study of the human prepubertal and pubertal larynx. Am J Anat 1978;151(1):11–9.

12. Wysocki J, Kielska E, Orszulak P, et al. Measurements of pre- and postpubertal human larynx: a cadaver study. Surg Radiol Anat 2008;30(3):191–9.

13. Litman RS, Weissend EE, Shibata D, et al. Developmental changes of laryngeal dimensions in unparalyzed, sedated children. Anesthesiology 2003;98(1):41–5.

14. Sprinzl GM, Eckel HE, Sittel C, et al. Morphometric measurements of the cartilaginous larynx: An anatomic correlate of laryngeal surgery. Head Neck 1999;21(8):743–50.

15. Standring S. Gray's anatomy: the anatomical basis of clinical practice. 42nd edition. Edinburgh: Elsevier; 2021.

16. Harries M, Hawkins S, Hacking J, et al. Changes in the male voice at puberty: vocal fold length and its relationship to the fundamental frequency of the voice. J Laryngol Otol 1998;112(5):451–4.

17. Amir O, Biron-Shental T. The impact of hormonal fluctuations on female vocal folds. Curr Opin Otolaryngol Head Neck Surg 2004;12(3):180–4.

18. Fitch WT, Giedd J. Morphology and development of the human vocal tract: a study using magnetic resonance imaging. J Acoust Soc Am 1999;106(3 Pt 1):1511–22.

19. Shaw RB, Katzel EB, Koltz PF, et al. Aging of the facial skeleton: aesthetic implications and rejuvenation strategies. Plast Reconstr Surg 2011;127(1):374–83.

20. Brown DL, Borschel GH, B L. Michigan manual of plastic surgery, vol. 2. Philadelphia, PA: Lippencott Williams & Wilkins (LLW); 2014.

21. Rohrich RJ, Avashia YJ, Savetsky IL. Prediction of facial aging using the facial fat compartments. Plast Reconstr Surg 2021;147(1S-2):38S–42S.

22. Shaw RB, Katzel EB, Koltz PF, et al. Aging of the mandible and its aesthetic implications. Plast Reconstr Surg 2010;125(1):332–42.

23. Coleman E, Radix AE, Bouman WP, et al. Standards of care for the health of transgender and gender diverse people, version 8. Int J Transgend Health 2022;23(Suppl 1):S1–259.

24. Chen K, Lu SM, Cheng R, et al. Facial recognition neural networks confirm success of facial feminization surgery. Plast Reconstr Surg 2020;145(1):203–9.

25. Fisher M, Lu SM, Chen K, et al. Facial feminization surgery changes perception of patient gender. Aesthet Surg J 2020;40(7):703–9.

26. Ainsworth TA, Spiegel JH. Quality of life of individuals with and without facial feminization surgery or gender reassignment surgery. Qual Life Res 2010;19(7):1019–24.

27. Morrison SD, Capitán-Cañadas F, Sánchez-García A, et al. Prospective quality-of-life outcomes after facial feminization surgery: an international multicenter study. Plast Reconstr Surg 2020;145(6):1499–509.

28. Getahun D, Nash R, Flanders WD, et al. Cross-sex hormones and acute cardiovascular events in transgender persons: a cohort study. Ann Intern Med 2018;169(4):205–13.

29. Coon D, Tuffaha S, Christensen J, et al. Reply: plastic surgery and smoking: a prospective analysis of incidence, compliance, and complications. Plast Reconstr Surg 2013;132(4):687e.

30. Rinker B. The evils of nicotine: an evidence-based guide to smoking and plastic surgery. Ann Plast Surg 2013;70(5):599–605.

31. Gutiérrez-Santamaría J, Simon D, Capitán L, et al. Shaping the lower jaw border with customized cutting guides: development, validation, and application in facial gender-affirming surgery. Facial Plast Surg Aesthet Med 2022. https://doi.org/10.1089/fpsam.2021.0418.

32. Canizares O, Thomson JE, Allen RJ, et al. The effect of processing technique on fat graft survival. Plast Reconstr Surg 2017;140(5):933–43.

33. Hanson SE, Garvey PB, Chang EI, et al. A prospective, randomized comparison of clinical outcomes with different processing techniques in autologous fat grafting. Plast Reconstr Surg 2022; 150(5):955–62.

34. Simon D, Capitán L, Bailón C, et al. Facial gender confirmation surgery: the lower jaw. description of surgical techniques and presentation of results. Plast Reconstr Surg 2022;149(4):755e–66e.

35. Park S, Lee TS. Strategic considerations for effective sagittal resection of the mandible to achieve a slim and attractive jawline. Plast Reconstr Surg 2018; 141(1):152–5.

36. Wu G, Xie Z, Shangguan W, et al. The accuracy of a patient-specific three-dimensional digital ostectomy template for mandibular angle ostectomy. Aesthet Surg J 2022;42(5):447–57.

37. Zhang C, Ma MW, Xu JJ, et al. Application of the 3D digital ostectomy template (DOT) in mandibular angle ostectomy (MAO). J Cranio-Maxillo-Fac Surg 2018;46(10):1821–7.

38. Kim NH, Park RH, Park JB. Botulinum toxin type A for the treatment of hypertrophy of the masseter muscle. Plast Reconstr Surg. Jun 2010;125(6): 1693–705.

39. Kundu N, Kothari R, Shah N, et al. Efficacy of botulinum toxin in masseter muscle hypertrophy for lower face contouring. J Cosmet Dermatol 2022;21(5):1849–56.

40. Tang CG, Debbaneh PM, Kleinberger AJ. Chondro-laryngoplasty. Otolaryngol Clin North Am 2022; 55(4):871–84.

41. Eggerstedt M, Lee JC, Mendelsohn AH. Transoral feminizing chondrolaryngoplasty: development and deployment of a novel approach in 77 patients. Facial Plast Surg Aesthet Med 2022. https://doi.org/10.1089/fpsam.2022.0016.

42. Raffaini M, Magri AS, Agostini T. Reply: full facial feminization surgery: patient satisfaction assessment based on 180 procedures involving 33 consecutive patients. Plast Reconstr Surg 2016; 138(4):766e–7e.

43. Gupta N, Wulu J, Spiegel JH. Safety of combined facial plastic procedures affecting multiple planes in a single setting in facial feminization for transgender patients. Aesthetic Plast Surg 2019;43(4): 993–9.

44. Morrison SD, Vyas KS, Motakef S, et al. Facial feminization: systematic review of the literature. Plast Reconstr Surg 2016;137(6):1759–70.

45. Telang PS. Facial feminization surgery: a review of 220 consecutive patients. Indian J Plast Surg 2020;53(2):244–53.

46. Caprini RM, Oberoi MK, Dejam D, et al. Effect of gender-affirming facial feminization surgery on psychosocial outcomes. Ann Surg 2022. https://doi.org/10.1097/SLA.0000000000005472.

Gender Affirming Facial Surgery–Anatomy and Procedures for Facial Masculinization

Arya Andre Akhavan, MD[a,b], John Henry Pang, MD[b],
Shane D. Morrison, MD[c], Thomas Satterwhite, MD[b,d],*

KEYWORDS

- Facial masculinization • Facial gender affirmation • Gender affirmation surgery

KEY POINTS

- The upper facial third can be masculinized via forehead and brow augmentation, and eyebrow augmentation and recontouring.
- The middle facial third can be masculinized via inferiolateral cheek augmentation, nasal masculinization/augmentation techniques, and orthognathic surgery.
- The lower facial third can be masculinized through numerous nonsurgical and surgical interventions, including orthognathic surgery of the chin and mandible, various fillers and implants, and thyroid cartilage augmentation.
- Patients may have different desired end-goals and testosterone exposure can variably masculinize different facial features, so each patient's surgical approach should be individualized.
- There are very few studies that specifically examine masculinizing procedures of the face specific to transgender men.

BACKGROUND

Gender affirmation surgery is a set of procedures that align a patient's physical characteristics with their identified gender. The human perception and social cognition literature has robustly shown that when humans view each other, the face is the first target of gaze, is a core feature of perception of gender, and can be the basis of many subconscious biases.[1] As a result, for some transgender men and nonbinary patients assigned female at birth, lack of masculine facial features may lead to misgendering by others, triggering dysphoria.[2] These patients may seek out facial masculinization surgery (FMS) to modify sexually-dimorphic facial structures, to produce a more masculine appearance.

The masculine and feminine faces are anatomically distinct (**Fig. 1**A–C). Broadly, the masculine face has an angular or M-shaped hairline, a wider forehead with prominent supraorbital ridge, a larger nose and mouth, and a square-shaped jaw with facial hair.[3–6] These features develop in response to testosterone exposure, as early as the prenatal period and potentially well into adulthood.[7] Patients seeking FMS may or may not have various components of these masculine facial characteristics, dependent on their personal hormonal exposure. Therefore, no single approach to FMS exists.

[a] Division of Plastic and Reconstructive Surgery, Rutgers New Jersey Medical School, 140 Bergen Street, Suite E1620, Newark, NJ 07103, USA; [b] Align Surgical Associates, 2299 Post Street, Suite 207, San Francisco, CA 94115, USA; [c] Division of Plastic Surgery, Department of Surgery, University of Washington School of Medicine, University of Washington, 1959 Northeast Pacific Street, Box 356165, Seattle, WA 98195, USA; [d] Division of Plastic and Reconstructive Surgery, Department of Surgery, Stanford University Medical Center
* Corresponding author.
E-mail address: tsatterwhite@alignsurgical.com

Oral Maxillofacial Surg Clin N Am 36 (2024) 221–236
https://doi.org/10.1016/j.coms.2024.01.001
1042-3699/24/© 2024 Elsevier Inc. All rights reserved.

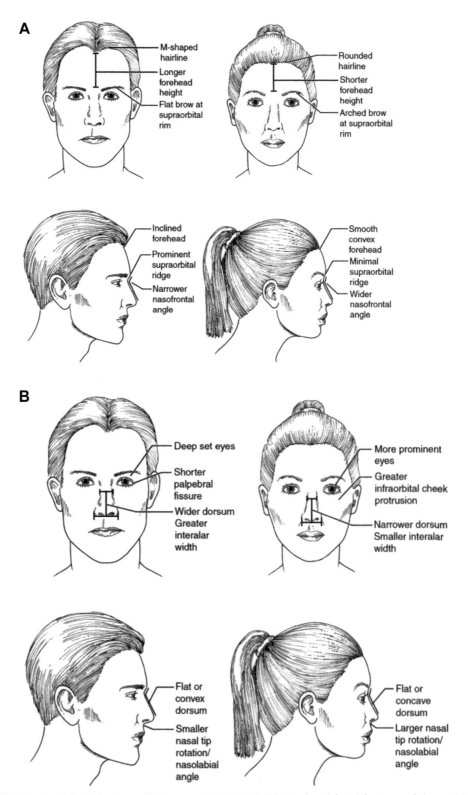

Fig. 1. (*A*) Gendered facial features of the upper facial third. (*B*) Gendered facial features of the middle facial third. (*C*) Gendered facial features of the lower facial third. (*From* Benjamin T, Knott PD, Seth R. Gender-affirming facial surgery: Anatomy and fundamentals of care. *Operative Techniques in Otolaryngology-Head and Neck Surgery.* 2023/03/01/ 2023;34(1):3-13. doi:https://doi.org/10.1016/j.otot.2023.01.002.)

C

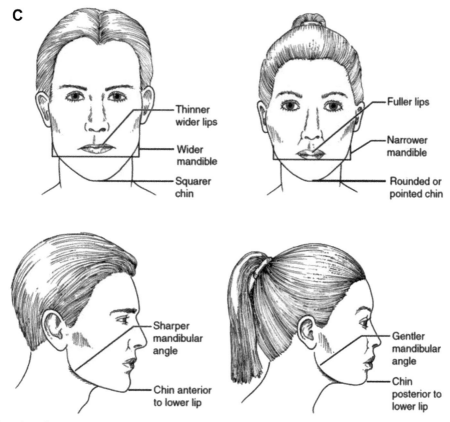

Thinner wider lips

Wider mandible

Squarer chin

Fuller lips

Narrower mandible

Rounded or pointed chin

Sharper mandibular angle

Chin anterior to lower lip

Gentler mandibular angle

Chin posterior to lower lip

Fig. 1. (continued)

FMS can vary from entirely nonsurgical, to panfacial reconstruction.[3,8,9] For patients with no prior testosterone exposure, medical facial masculinization via testosterone therapy has been shown to increase the width of the jaw and decrease the width of the cheeks.[10,11] It also variably induces facial hair growth, which is masculinizing and often highly desirable for patients, and can induce androgenic alopecia, which can be masculinizing, but may or may not be desirable.[12,13]

This article will discuss procedural and surgical facial masculinization. The vertical facial thirds will be reviewed, with a description of anatomic sexual dimorphism followed by FMS techniques.

THE UPPER FACIAL THIRD—HAIRLINE, FOREHEAD, AND BROW
Anatomy

The upper facial third includes the hairline, foreheadand brow, and eyebrow, which are salient indicators of masculinity.[4–6,14,15] The male hairline is higher than that of women, with more prominent lateral recessions creating an "M" shape.[16] This higher hairline with lateral recessions leads to a taller, wider-appearing forehead than in women.[17]

The brow is more prominent, with a stronger supracillary ridge and supraorbital bossing. The masculine eyebrow is straighter and directly on the supracillary ridge, while feminine eyebrows are typically peaked at the lateral third and lie above the supracillary ridge.

Procedures

Hairline masculinization
Surgical and nonsurgical techniques for hairline masculinization have not been described in transgender men and are unlikely to be sought. Testosterone therapy is usually sufficient to induce male-pattern hairline changes in transgender men, though this varies between individuals. While a receding hairline is masculinizing, it is generally considered unaesthetic. If a patient desires hairline recession, then depilation techniques may be considered, including laser hair removal or electrolytic depilation.

Forehead and brow masculinization
The forehead-brow region is a prominent gender marker,[18] with an appearance almost wholly dependent on the underlying native bone.

Masculinization of the forehead requires an increase in volume to the bony architecture, as well as curvature changes (**Fig. 2**).

Filler-based or fat graft-based augmentation is often insufficient. Injections and grafts are used to add malleable volume; however, the thick inelastic overlying skin and frontalis muscle tonicity prevent substantial volume gain, and may lead to material spreading from the target site. Botulinum injection into the frontalis muscle 4 weeks prior can loosen the muscular soft tissue envelope and facilitate filler placement.[19] Mild nonsurgical brow augmentation may be achieved with filler injection from the brow tail to the frontal protuberance.[19]

Fat grafts are more permanent, but immediate postoperative absorption is variable and may lead to soft tissue heterogeneity. Both fat grafting and fillers carry risk of embolic events to the ophthalmic artery during injection, via high-pressure retrograde flow through anastomoses to the supraorbital and supratrochlear artery. The literature describes numerous cases of blindness after injections to the forehead, brow, and glabella, which can be partially reversed if hyaluronic acid fillers were used but cannot be reversed if fat grafting was performed.[20–22] As such, surgeons should carefully consider and discuss the benefits, risks, and limitations of filler and fat grafting of the upper third with patients.

On the other hand, open surgical approaches to forehead masculinization can directly augment the area with permanent firm material (**Fig. 3**). Multiple options exist, including synthetic non-absorbable materials, exogenous acellular bony scaffolding, and autogenous bone grafting. Placement of these materials requires an open approach. However, evidence for each of these interventions is limited by small sample sizes.[17,23–26]

Autologous bone grafting has been reported. Split-calvarial bone grafting produces appropriate native bone for frontal augmentation, but requires a second surgical site. In addition, the split calvarial bone harvest technique carries with it unpredictable rates of bony resorption after grafting,[27] and some patients may not have a truly bicortical calvarium, increasing risk of dural violation. Other autogenous options include the iliac crest and rib, but come with additional donor site morbidity and unpredictable rates of bony resorption. Fixation of the grafts also requires hardware which can cause contour deformity and can increase infection risks.

Eyebrow masculinization

Multiple nonsurgical, minimally-invasive, and open techniques exist for masculinization of the eyebrow, and follow principles similar to those for aesthetic changes to the eyebrow as well as eyebrow reconstruction.

Principles of frontalis chemodenervation for eyebrow feminization can be reversed to cause masculinization. Botulinum can be placed above the brow arch in the frontalis muscle belly, to drop the feminine arch of the eyebrow and produce a flatter, more masculine appearance.[28] Injecting the far lateral brow can drop the brow onto the supraciliary ridge, again for a more masculine appearance.[29] However, in patients with compensated blepharoptosis who rely on frontalis activation as an upper eyelid elevator, caution must be used to avoid vision-compromising brow and upper lid ptosis.[28] Similarly, excess placement in the lateral brow can cause vision-obscuring hooding.

Hair transplantation is a well-known technique for eyebrow reconstruction in burns, and has been described for eyebrow enhancement.[30] Follicular unit extraction is performed, typically using the occipital scalp but potentially using other sites that have responded to testosterone (**Fig. 4**).[31] Selected 1-shaft or 2-shaft follicular units are placed at an angle to mimic natural eyebrow growth, and are used to thicken and

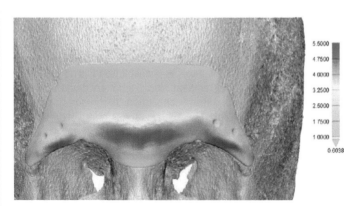

Fig. 2. Contour mapping in frontal augmentation.

5.5000
4.7500
4.0000
3.2500
2.5000
1.7500
1.0000
0.0038

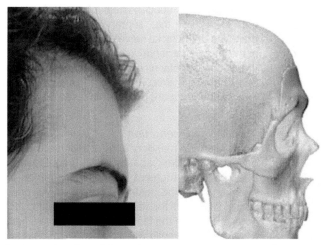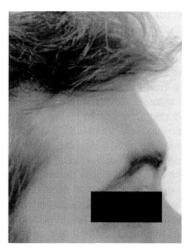

Fig. 3. Implant-based frontal augmentation using virtual surgical planning (VSP) methods.

lower the eyebrow, and decrease lateral peaking. Follicular unit transplantation includes additional donor site morbidity and scarring but does not require shaving the head. Patients must be counseled about eyebrow trimming and thickness limitations, as hair follicles of scalp origin have a longer anagen phase and narrower diameter. Limited studies on eyebrow transplantation suggest patient satisfaction and good cosmesis.[32]

THE MIDDLE FACIAL THIRD—THE NOSE, MALAR REGION, AND MAXILLA
Anatomy

The middle facial third includes the nose, the malar region, and the maxilla, with the nose providing the strongest gendered features. The masculine nose features a wider nasal bony pyramid and more acute nasofrontal angle due to frontal bossing. The masculine nose also has a straight or convex dorsal contour with or without a dorsal hump, as compared to the convex-to-straight feminine nose. Finally, the masculine nasal tip has a more acute nasolabial angle, without a supratip break.[33–36]

The malar region demonstrates sexual dimorphism in both the projection and contour of the

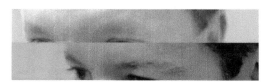

Fig. 4. Eyebrow augmentation via transplant, using testosterone-responsive leg hair. (*From* Umar S. Eyebrow transplantation: Alternative body sites as a donor source. *Journal of the American Academy of Dermatology.* 2014/10/01/ 2014;71(4):e140-e141.)

zygomatic bone, and in overlying facial fat pad suspension and distribution. The male cheek is fuller anteromedially, with a laterally larger and clockwise-rotated zygomatic bone, creating the appearance of a broader, flatter cheek. In contrast, women have increased anterior fat pad volume and a narrower zygomatic bone, creating a rounder cheek.[37] The cheeks are modestly affected by hormone therapy in transgender men, with a decrease in width of about half a millimeter after a year of testosterone.[10] The zygomatic branches of the facial nerve run under the zygomaticus muscle, and may be encountered during deep dissection (see *Malar Masculinization*).

The interplay of the size, projection, and width of the maxilla compared to the zygomatic bone can influence the perceived size and shape of the zygoma. Similarly, the interplay of the maxilla, piriform aperture, and nose can alter the perception of nasal projection and width. In general, the masculine midface is characterized by a wide and anteriorly positioned maxilla, with the maxilla and upper dentition providing prominent lip support.

Procedures

Nasal masculinization
Masculinizing rhinoplasty has been described for cisgender men, but is rarely described specifically for gender affirmation.[17,38] Principles remain similar to those performed in cisgender men, which generally involve augmentation, but may require more volume in transgender patients. Both nonsurgical injections and open surgical techniques with grafting can be successful.

Nonsurgical "liquid" rhinoplasty via filler injection may be sufficient when modest or temporary changes are desired.[39] Liquid rhinoplasty features similar risk of ophthalmic artery embolism and blindness via the dorsal nasal artery or other adjacent vessels, and high-pressure injection to the nasal tip may lead to skin ischemia and necrosis.[20–22,40] Due to particular vascular sensitivity of the nasal skin, skin color and texture should be monitored closely during injection. Deep supraperichondrial or immediate supraperiosteal injection on withdrawal decreases risk. For nasal widening, filler is injected at the junction of bony dorsum and lateral nasal bone.[41] For the nasal dorsum, filler should be threaded along the long axis of the dorsum to preserve contour.[41,42] For the nasal sidewall, cross-hatched small-volume placement can achieve uniform augmentation. For the nasal tip and ala, serial punctures with very small volumes will both allow for finer volume control and contour, and to help reduce the risk of skin necrosis.[42]

In open augmentation rhinoplasty, cartilage grafting can provide larger, permanent volume changes. Grafts may be taken from the concha or from rib cartilage. Septal cartilage may be considered, but over-resection should be carefully avoided. Feminine dorsal concavity can be corrected with dorsal onlay grafts, or spreader grafts can be used to concurrently alter the dorsum and provide widening.[34] Nasal tip lengthening, clockwise rotation, and augmentation can similarly be performed with various combinations of tip cap or shield grafts, columellar strut grafts, and extension grafts. However, care must be taken to avoid excessive reduction or tip refinement, which may be feminizing.[34]

Malar augmentation

Nonsurgical and surgical masculinization of the malar region is infrequently described. The cheeks can be augmented with both facial fillers and fat grafting superficially, and structural fillers may be injected subperiosteally.[43] However, care must be taken not to fill the anteriomedial compartment as increased anterior projection creates a feminized appearance, and should instead be focused inferiolaterally to increase cheek width, not projection.[43]

Facial implants for malar masculinization are similarly underreported, though some orthognathic and reconstructive surgery literature is present for midface hypoplasia.[44] Implants can be placed through an intraoral approach, which hides visible scars but increases the risk for implant infection, or can be placed through periorbital or facelift incisions, with external scarring visible but lower infection risk.[45] Other risks include bone resorption underneath the implant, as well as soft tissue malposition overlying the implant. Implants should be placed in a subperiosteal plane, taking care not to injure the supraperiosteal zygomatic branches of the facial nerve during all approaches, or the infraorbital nerve during intraoral approach.[45] Virtual surgical planning (VSP) may similarly be of benefit during malar/zygomatic implant placement to provide for a more predictable result (**Fig. 5**).

Maxillary augmentation

Facial fillers for maxillary augmentation are poorly described. Hydroxyapatite (HA) granules have been used to augment the maxillary region for reconstructive and aesthetic purposes. As previously discussed for forehead augmentation, HA augmentation of the facial skeleton can yield highly satisfactory results with low complication rates. For maxillary augmentation, an intraoral incision is used to gain access to the maxilla, and HA crystals are placed subperiosteally at the superior border of the maxilla, or in other areas where augmentation is desired.[27]

The best-described maxillary augmentation, the LeFort 1 advancement (with or without occlusal plane rotation), has not been studied as a masculinizing procedure in gender affirmation. LeFort 1 advancements are typically performed in an orthognathic context, usually require orthodontic braces, and are rarely covered by insurance even when medically necessary.[46] The changes associated with maxillary advancement carry a mixed masculinizing-feminizing picture. LeFort 1 advancement augments the anteriomedial cheek more than inferiolaterally, which may be feminizing to a degree.[47] In the perioral region, maxillary advancement provides strongly increased bony and dental support to the upper lip, both of which are masculinizing.[48] And in the nasal region, maxillary advancement causes anterior displacement of the inferior border of the piriform aperture, with an accompanying masculinizing increase in nasal

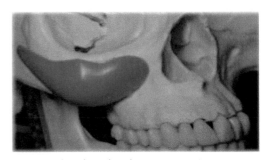

Fig. 5. Implant-based malar augmentation using VSP methods. (*From* Livieri P, Uribe FA, Quereshy FA. Aesthetic Facial Surgery and Orthodontics: Common Goals. Oral and maxillofacial surgery clinics of North America. 2020/02/01/ 2020;32(1):153-165.)

projection and alar width, but also causes a feminizing increase in nasolabial angle.[49]

Other orthognathic procedures can also achieve masculinization of the midface.[50] Counterclockwise rotation of the maxillomandibular complex can widen the alar base, philtrum, and oral width, increase lip projection, decrease tooth show both at rest and when smiling, and advance the chin point (see *Chin Augmentation*).[49,51,52] All of these effects are masculinizing. Surgical planning of orthognathic procedures for gender affirmation should include orthodontic specialists to ensure maintenance of occlusion or correction of malocclusion.

THE LOWER FACIAL THIRD—THE MOUTH, MANDIBLE, CHIN, AND NECK
Anatomy

The lower facial third consists of the lower jaw, mouth, and chin; thyroid cartilage (Adam's apple), and facial hair. Given that this area is one of the strongest facial indicators of gender, masculinization of this region has comparatively high yield.[4]

The mandible, chin, and mouth can be considered as a single unit, can all be approached in the same procedure, and changes to one site impact the others. The masculine mandible is more prominent in multiple aspects.[53] A more acute mandibular angle and greater transverse gonial splay lead to a square shape on anterior view.[54,55] The base of the mandible is wider in men than in women, with the lateral projection of the mandible extending approximately to the lateral projection of the zygoma.[56] The chin can be considered as a distinct subzone; it is higher, broader, and wider in men than in women, and has greater projection and lateral bulk.[17] The mouth in men is typically wider than in women, with thinner lips, a longer philtrum, less maxillary tooth show, and decreased vermillion show.[54,55]

The lower face and neck also include facial hair and the thyroid cartilage. The size and prominence of the thyroid cartilage ("Adam's apple") is strongly linked to masculinity, with a larger, more angular, and more anteriorly projected thyroid cartilage in men.[57,58] In addition, dense facial hair, particularly large beards with high hair density, is a strongly masculinizing feature.[59] Patients seeking facial masculinization often strongly desire facial hair development, regardless of preferred style.[60]

Procedures

Mandibular augmentation
Testosterone supplementation causes noninvasive mandibular augmentation (predominantly widening).[10] Mandibular augmentation with fillers

can create a stronger appearing, squarer jaw.[61] Fillers may be injected from an intra-oral approach lateral to the second premolar, avoiding the mental foramen, and administered via small aliquots in a retrograde fanning pattern.[19,43] Use of hyaluronic acid, hydroxyapatite, and poly-L-lactic acid have all been described.[19,62,63] The choice to use compressible or incompressible filler depends on skin thickness and pre-procedural mandibular definition.[62]

Fat grafting may be performed, but there are no standardized techniques for the mandible; volume should be determined on a patient-dependent basis. Fine cannulas may help prevent contour irregularities and ensure even distribution.[61] Fat grafting to the perimandibular soft tissue should remain superficial and above the inferior border of the mandible, to avoid injury to critical neurovascular structures. Compared to soft tissue fillers, resorption rates in fat grafting are unpredictable.[64]

Surgical mandibular augmentation is typically done through intraoral incisions, and can be achieved via synthetic, scaffold, or bone implantation (**Fig. 6**). Porous implants allow bony ingrowth and are easier to surgically manipulate, but bony ingrowth means they are more difficult to remove if infected.[17] Patients report high satisfaction and few complications.[17] In contrast, silicone implants are more difficult to manipulate surgically, but are less likely to become infected and are easier to remove in the setting of infection.[65]

Hydroxyapatite granules can also augment the mandible with generally high aesthetic satisfaction.[27] However, complications of hydroxyapatite appear to be more prevalent in the mandible. The mandible is especially susceptible to contour irregularity, infection, granule extrusion, and seroma.[27] Autogenous bone grafts may also add mandibular bulk, but have high rates of bony resorption.[17,66] Autogenous bone grafts may be calvarial or iliac in origin, and can provide mandibular widening and a more acute gonial angle with good patient satisfaction when placed between the medial two-thirds and lateral one-third of the mandible above the pterygomasseteric fascial sling.[17,67]

Mandibular augmentation can also be achieved via orthognathic surgery (**Fig. 7**).[68] Bilateral sagittal split osteotomies allow for anterioposterior and rotational changes. Mandibular advancement itself masculinizes the facial profile and augments the mandibular width and angle, while occlusal plane changes via rotation may also be masculinizing.[69–71]

Chin augmentation
Chin augmentation can be achieved through multiple methods. Filler placement and fat grafting

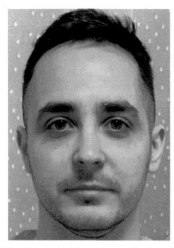
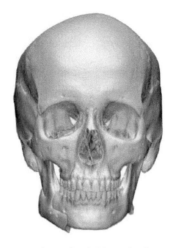
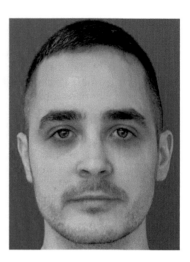

Fig. 6. Implant-based mandibular augmentation using VSP methods.

allow for customizable 3D chin augmentation without visible incisions or scarring.[19,43,72–74] Botulinum toxin injection 2 weeks prior can loosen the skin envelope and facilitate injection of filler,[63] and fillers may be placed either in the subcutaneous and deep adipose layers, or deep to the mentalis muscle centrally.[9,19] Techniques for fat grafting to the chin follow the same guidelines, and considerations are largely similar to fat grafting in other facial regions.

Chin implants are common in cisgender patients, effectively increase anterior projection, and are increasingly customizable.[75] They are placed via intraoral or submental incisions, with intraoral incisions avoiding visible scarring at the cost of increased infection risk. Implants may be placed in a subperiosteal, supraperiosteal, or mixed plane, with the subperiosteal location allowing for the best fixation at the cost of possible mandibular erosion. Mixed-plane techniques with supraperiosteal central placement and subperiosteal lateral placement allow increase fixation laterally and avoidance of central erosion. Complications include malpositioning and migration, although these may be mitigated by reapproximation of the mentalis muscle and use of postoperative compression dressings.[75]

Osseous genioplasty provides durable masculinizing chin augmentation, and may be more customizable than implants[17] (**Fig. 8**). An axial osteotomy is performed and the chin is distracted anteriorly. Vertical split, transverse distraction, and rotation provide further customization, and residual spaces can be filled with bone grafts, hydroxyapatite granules, and other bony growth agents. Cisgender patients report high satisfaction with comparatively few complications, though mental nerve injury and malunion have been reported.[75]

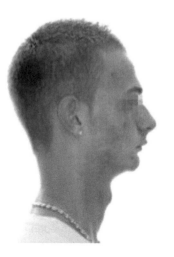
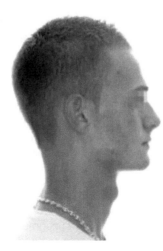

Fig. 7. Mandibular advancement with resulting masculinization. (Reproduced from Olivi P, Garcia C. Bi-maxillary advancement surgery: Technique, indications and results. International Orthodontics. 2014/06/01/ 2014;12(2):200-212. Copyright © 2014 Elsevier Masson SAS. All rights reserved.)

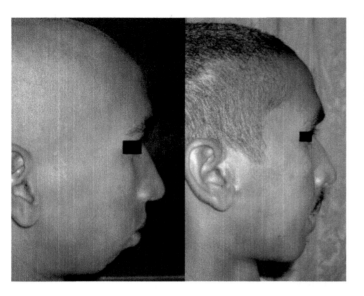

Fig. 8. Sliding osseous genioplasty with resulting masculinization. (*From* Singh S, Mehrotra D, Mohammad S. Profile changes after conventional and chin shield genioplasty. Journal of Oral Biology and Craniofacial Research. 2014/05/01/ 2014;4(2):70-75.)

Upper lip reduction and oral widening

Multiple reconstructive and aesthetic procedures of the mouth and lips are applicable to facial masculinization, though they have not been described in the FMS context. Use of fillers to augment the lips is feminizing and unlikely to be desired.[43] Reduction of upper lip vermilion and lengthening of the philtrum via vermillion reduction cheiloplasty has been described in primarily nonwhite cisgender patients.[76] This technique requires careful design of the modified ellipses to be excised, as to not obliterate cupid's bow.[77] Oral commissuroplasty techniques for microstomia can be applied to FMS to widen the mouth, though this has not been described.

Thyroid cartilage augmentation

Thyroid cartilage augmentation is strongly masculinizing, but rarely described in the literature. Androgen exposure during puberty leads to thyroid cartilage growth, but literature on postpubertal testosterone exposure is absent.[78] Thyroid cartilage augmentation with rib cartilage grafts has been described specifically for FMS. In a report, a pyramid-shaped graft was placed in a subperichondrial position through a submental incision, adhering directly to the thyroid cartilage.[79] Possible complications include injury to the larynx and laryngeal nerve. There are no current reports of implant use or other augmentation methods.

Facial hair augmentation

Facial hair can be achieved through hormone therapy alone. In fact, patients may have ongoing robust facial hair development over a multi-year period as they continue on testosterone supplementation.[80] Patients who desire further facial hair growth without surgical intervention may consider topical agents used for androgenetic alopecia, such as minoxidil.[81]

Some patients may not respond to medical therapy, and may consider facial hair transplant (**Fig. 9**).[60,82] Transgender men have less dense and shorter hair at donor sites than cisgender men, which may differ from native facial hair that arises from testosterone therapy.[83] As with any facial hair transplant, small grafts and recipient sites, angled as close to the skin as possible, will provide for a more natural appearance.[60]

IMPLANTABLE MATERIALS
Augmentation Materials

Polymethylmethacrylate (MMA) is a nonabsorbable malleable polymer that is mixed intraoperatively and applied directly to the site.[23–26] Unlike other materials, MMA is malleable before curing, allowing in-field customization, and can be placed with or without bony fixation. However, MMA cures exothermically, reaching up to 82°C (180°F), and can cause thermal bone necrosis.[23] This must be prevented by active cooled irrigation during curing. While data on MMA use in FMS are limited, patients show high satisfaction and suffer only minor complications such as seroma.[17,25]

In contrast, preformed implants do not require molding, curing, or cooling. Polyether ether ketone (PEEK) is an organic polymer with similar mechanical properties to bone.[84] It is well described in facial reconstruction and facial

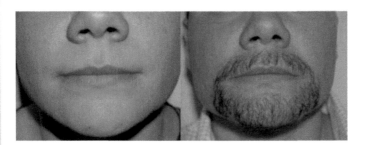

Fig. 9. Beard augmentation via transplant, using occipital hair. (*From* Epstein J, Bared A. Gender-affirming hair procedures. Operative Techniques in Otolaryngology-Head and Neck Surgery. 2023/03/01/ 2023;34(1):19-29.)

aesthetics.[85–87] While a substantial number of off-the-shelf components exist, which can be burred for customization, PEEK is often pre-milled with computer-aided design (CAD)/computer-aided manufacturing (CAM) techniques and custom fixators. Its use offers predictable results with good patient satisfaction.[88,89] Porous polyethylene (PPE) products are related to PEEK, but offer slightly different properties. PPE implants are softer and can be shaped with a blade, but can still be fixated directly to bone.[90] The porosity of the surface allows for soft tissue ingrowth, which has been reported to reduce infections rates, but ingrowth causes a more difficult explantation if complications arise.[91] Animal models also show reasonable safety in PPE laryngotracheoplasty, suggesting possible use in tracheal augmentation.[92] Silicone facial implants are generally the softest and can similarly be placed in a dissected pocket without bony fixation.[93] In contrast to PEEK and PPE, silicone implants can have variable firmness and can be used to augment cartilaginous areas, such as the nose.[94] All of the above products are associated with some degree of long-term bony resorption at the placement site, as well as risk of infection.[90]

Calcium-deficient HA is the primary component of native bone by mass, and has been used as bony scaffolding matrix for over 30 years—including augmentation of the calvarium and mandible.[95,96] As a volumizing osteointegrative scaffolding material, its predominant advantages are the lack of risks associated with foreign bodies, and the lack of bone resorption at the placement site.[17,27] The material is typically placed as porous granules in a subperiosteal plane, with some non-FMS literature recommending superficial corticotomy to accelerate osteointegration. The material can be inadvertently compacted, causing volume loss, and can be resorbed rather than integrated, with variable absorption rates reported.[97] Evidence for its use is limited for FMS, though satisfactory cosmesis (96%) and low complication rates have been reported.[27]

DISCUSSION
Current State and Future Directions

Facial masculinization surgery is relatively uncommon.[98] Some patients may not seek facial masculinization due to lack of a perceived need. Others may be content with the facial masculinizing effects of testosterone therapy and may not desire further intervention.[10–13] The reasons for facial masculinization's low prevalence have not been studied, but may be attributable to greater salience of masculine facial features versus feminine ones, or the lower rates of men seeking cosmetic surgery versus women. Another possibility is that the range of "acceptable" masculine facial characteristics is broader, compared to the narrow rigid definitions of facial femininity. Thus, transgender men with less-masculine features may be scrutinized less, as compared to transgender women with less-feminine features.

While currently uncommon, facial masculinization is likely to increase in prevalence. Increased training of plastic surgeons around gender-affirming surgery procedures, with the institution of multiple new gender affirmation surgical fellowships, will likely increase long-term patient access.

Technological and Material Advances

Implantable materials are rapidly advancing. The variety of materials, and available sizes and shapes of preformed products, has greatly increased, and research is being targeted toward new materials designed ab initio for specific properties, such as biocompatibility and incorporation into native tissue. Advances in 3D printing and VSP have led to custom augmenting implants made of PEEK and various calcium products used in reconstructive surgery, and cutting guides used to aid in orthognathic surgery.[99–101] These are now being applied to masculinizing facial surgery, though little published research exists specifically describing the use of 3D printing in gender affirmation. While these techniques offer a much greater degree of customization and predictability, they are costly, and most off-the-shelf products can be shaped with burrs. The cost/benefit tradeoff should be discussed with patients.

Patient Variability and Trade-offs

Patients seeking facial masculinization may have dramatically different interventional needs, dependent on natal, pubertal, and postpubertal hormone exposure; individual goals; and degree of dysphoria over specific facial features.

Nonsurgical treatments are less expensive and can be associated with lower overall risk. Their impermanence is both a flaw and a feature, as patients can perform "trial runs" to determine their preferred areas for augmentation. Some patients prefer to use only nonsurgical treatments, while others may then "convert" to surgical intervention. Surgeons should be aware of prior history of nonsurgical treatment, as repeated panfacial injections may lead to complications such as granuloma formation[102] and may increase subsequent difficulty of facial surgery.[103] However, prior nonsurgical treatment should not preclude future surgery.[9]

Additional potential trade-offs exist. Many cosmetic procedures for facial rejuvenation in cisgender men have partially feminizing effects. These should be used with caution in transgender men who may wish to avoid feminization of any kind. For example, botulinum for "crow's feet" or glabellar-corrugator rhytids may concurrently achieve facial rejuvenation by reducing wrinkles, and also raise the brow and create feminization. Therefore, patient preferences should be considered individually.

Special Considerations for Non-binary and Non-white Patients

The gender affirmation goals of nonbinary patients assigned female at birth may vary considerably from those of transgender men. Priorities of nonbinary patients seeking facial masculinization have not been explicitly studied. However, differential priorities between non-binary patients and transgender men have been documented in other types of gender-affirming surgeries,[104,105] and it is certainly possible that these differences may apply to facial masculinization.

In addition, patient anatomy and goals may vary by ethnoracial and cultural background. In cisgender patients, the so-called "ethnic rhinoplasty" refers to a broad set of techniques that can be applied to non-Caucasian rhinoplasty to maintain certain ethnic features,[106,107] and some more recent literature now examines procedures on an individual ethnic group basis.[108] Patients seeking facial masculinization may have ethnoracial or cultural preferences for anatomic end-goals. As these data are lacking in the facial masculinization literature, application of relevant literature in cisgender patients will likely be fruitful.[76,109–114]

Limitations of Current Data

There is a significant lack of data on masculinizing facial procedures as specifically performed in transgender and gender-diverse patients. This limits our understanding of the impact of hormone therapy on facial structure, as well as clinical outcomes and patient-reported outcomes associated with nonsurgical treatments and masculinizing surgery, preventing the development of concrete guidelines. Given this lack of data, surgeons may use masculinizing procedures designed for cisgender patients.

Substantial further research is needed. Thankfully, with a large number of active research groups contributing to the literature, more concrete data are forthcoming.

CLINICS CARE POINTS

- Hairline, Forehead, and Brow Masculinization
  - Pearls
    - An open-approach placement of a synthetic, patient-tailored forehead construct is a highly effective masculinizing technique of the upper third of the face
    - Targeted chemodenervation of the frontalis can drop portions of the brow to create a less arched, lower, more masculine appearance
    - Hair transplantation is effective to thicken and masculinize the brow
  - Pitfalls
    - Exogenous testosterone masculinizes the hairline but may lead to dys-aesthetic thinning and recession
    - Facial fillers for forehead and brow masculinization are likely to migrate, and the tissues are unlikely to accept enough volume for significant changes
    - If using polymethylmethacrylate, failure to constantly cure the material can cause thermal injury to the patient
- Nose, Cheek, and Maxilla Masculinization
  - Pearls
    - Open rhinoplasty is highly effective at masculinizing the face, particularly with

attention to augmentation with rib/conchal cartilage, and masculinizing maneuvers such as clockwise rotation and tip lengthening

- Structural subperiosteal filler, placed inferiolaterally can effectively masculinize the cheeks without open surgical intervention
- Orthognathic surgery of the maxilla is a highly effective, multidimensional technique for dramatic masculinization of the midface

  o Pitfalls

- Nasal augmentation with filler requires care to avoid intravascular injection and potential severe complications including blindness
- Misplacement of cheek filler in a superiomedial position over the zygoma can inadvertently feminize the face

- Mandible and Chin Masculinization

  o Pearls

- Orthognathic surgery, particularly mandibular advancement with sliding genioplasty, is a highly effective, multidimensional technique for dramatic masculinization of the jawline
- Facial fillers can be a powerful adjunct for facial masculinization, particularly for the mandibular and gonial angles

  o Pitfalls

- Fat grafting for mandibular augmentation has unpredictable resorption rates
- Autogenous bone grafts have high rates of absorption when used for mandibular augmentation

- Additional Masculinizing Techniques

  o Pearls

- Facial hair growth is often successful with nonsurgical adjuncts, such as exogenous testosterone and topical minoxidil

  o Pitfalls

- Thyroid cartilage augmentation is rarely reported and carries risk of nerve injury

DISCLOSURE

The authors have nothing to disclose.

REFERENCES

1. Hadders-Algra M. Human face and gaze perception is highly context specific and involves bottom-up and top-down neural processing. Neurosci Biobehav Rev 2022;132:304–23.
2. Oles N, Darrach H, Landford W, et al. Gender Affirming Surgery: A Comprehensive, Systematic Review of All Peer-reviewed Literature and Methods of Assessing Patient-centered Outcomes (Part 1: Breast/Chest, Face, and Voice). Ann Surg 2022;275(1):e52–66.
3. Sayegh F, Ludwig DC, Ascha M, et al. Facial Masculinization Surgery and its Role in the Treatment of Gender Dysphoria. J Craniofac Surg 2019;30(5):1339–46.
4. Brown E, Perrett DI. What gives a face its gender? Perception 1993;22(7):829–40.
5. Roberts T, Bruce V. Feature saliency in judging the sex and familiarity of faces. Perception 1988;17(4):475–81.
6. Bruce V, Burton AM, Hanna E, et al. Sex discrimination: how do we tell the difference between male and female faces? Perception 1993;22(2):131–52.
7. Whitehouse AJ, Gilani SZ, Shafait F, et al. Prenatal testosterone exposure is related to sexually dimorphic facial morphology in adulthood. Proc Biol Sci 2015;282(1816):20151351.
8. Morrison SD, Satterwhite T. Lower Jaw Recontouring in Facial Gender-Affirming Surgery. Facial plastic surgery clinics of North America 2019;27(2):233–42.
9. Ascha M, Swanson MA, Massie JP, et al. Nonsurgical Management of Facial Masculinization and Feminization. Aesthetic Surg J 2019;39(5):Np123–37.
10. Tebbens M, Nota NM, Liberton N, et al. Gender-Affirming Hormone Treatment Induces Facial Feminization in Transwomen and Masculinization in Transmen: Quantification by 3D Scanning and Patient-Reported Outcome Measures. J Sex Med 2019;16(5):746–54.
11. Hembree WC, Cohen-Kettenis P, Delemarre-van de Waal HA, et al. Endocrine treatment of transsexual persons: an Endocrine Society clinical practice guideline. J Clin Endocrinol Metab 2009;94(9):3132–54.
12. Van Caenegem E, Wierckx K, Taes Y, et al. Body composition, bone turnover, and bone mass in trans men during testosterone treatment: 1-year follow-up data from a prospective case-controlled study (ENIGI). Eur J Endocrinol 2015;172(2):163–71.
13. Dhingra N, Bonati LM, Wang EB, et al. Medical and aesthetic procedural dermatology recommendations for transgender patients undergoing transition. J Am Acad Dermatol 2019;80(6):1712–21.
14. Spiegel JH. Facial determinants of female gender and feminizing forehead cranioplasty. Laryngoscope 2011;121(2):250–61.

15. Ousterhout DK. Feminization of the forehead: contour changing to improve female aesthetics. Plast Reconstr Surg 1987;79(5):701–13.

16. Nusbaum BP, Fuentefria S. Naturally occurring female hairline patterns. Dermatol Surg 2009;35(6): 907–13.

17. Ousterhout DK. Dr. Paul Tessier and facial skeletal masculinization. Ann Plast Surg 2011;67(6):S10–5.

18. Deschamps-Braly JC. Approach to Feminization Surgery and Facial Masculinization Surgery: Aesthetic Goals and Principles of Management. J Craniofac Surg 2019;30(5):1352–8.

19. Scherer MA. Specific aspects of a combined approach to male face correction: botulinum toxin A and volumetric fillers. J Cosmet Dermatol 2016; 15(4):566–74.

20. Zhang L, Pan L, Xu H, et al. Clinical Observations and the Anatomical Basis of Blindness After Facial Hyaluronic Acid Injection. Aesthetic Plast Surg 2019;43(4):1054–60.

21. Li X, Du L, Lu JJ. A Novel Hypothesis of Visual Loss Secondary to Cosmetic Facial Filler Injection. Ann Plast Surg 2015;75(3):258–60.

22. Wu S, Pan L, Wu H, et al. Anatomic Study of Ophthalmic Artery Embolism Following Cosmetic Injection. Journal of Craniofacial Surgery Sep 2017;28(6):1578–81.

23. Stelnicki EJ, Ousterhout DK. Prevention of thermal tissue injury induced by the application of polymethylmethacrylate to the calvarium. J Craniofac Surg 1996;7(3):192–5.

24. Ousterhout DK, Baker S, Zlotolow I. Methylmethacrylate onlay implants in the treatment of forehead deformities secondary to craniosynostosis. J Maxillofac Surg 1980;8(3):228–33.

25. Ousterhout DK, Zlotolow IM. Aesthetic improvement of the forehead utilizing methylmethacrylate onlay implants. Aesthetic Plastic Surgery Fall 1990;14(4):281–5.

26. Marchac D, Greensmith A. Long-term experience with methylmethacrylate cranioplasty in craniofacial surgery. J Plast Reconstr Aesthetic Surg 2008;61(7):744–52. discussion 753.

27. Moreira-Gonzalez A, Jackson IT, Miyawaki T, et al. Augmentation of the craniomaxillofacial region using porous hydroxyapatite granules. Plast Reconstr Surg 2003;111(6):1808–17.

28. Flynn TC. Botox in men. Dermatol Ther 2007;20(6): 407–13.

29. Cohen BE, Bashey S, Wysong A. Literature review of cosmetic procedures in men: approaches and techniques are gender specific. Am J Clin Dermatol 2017;18(1):87–96.

30. Tomc CM, Malouf PJ. Eyebrow restoration: the approach, considerations, and technique in follicular unit transplantation. J Cosmet Dermatol 2015; 14(4):310–4.

31. Umar S. Eyebrow transplantation: Alternative body sites as a donor source. J Am Acad Dermatol 2014; 71(4):e140–1.

32. Bared A, Epstein JS. Gender-affirmation hair transplantation techniques. Facial Plastic Surgery clinics of North America 2023;31(3):375–80.

33. Chronicle EP, Chan MY, Hawkings C, et al. You can tell by the nose–judging sex from an isolated facial feature. Perception 1995;24(8):969–73.

34. Rohrich RJ, Janis JE, Kenkel JM. Male rhinoplasty. Plast Reconstr Surg 2003;112(4):1071–85. quiz 1086.

35. Mitteroecker P, Windhager S, Muller GB, et al. The morphometrics of "masculinity" in human faces. PLoS One 2015;10(2):e0118374.

36. Hage JJ, Becking AG, de Graaf FH, et al. Gender-confirming facial surgery: considerations on the masculinity and femininity of faces. Plast Reconstr Surg 1997;99(7):1799–807.

37. Koudelova J, Bruzek J, Caganova V, et al. Development of facial sexual dimorphism in children aged between 12 and 15 years: a three-dimensional longitudinal study. Orthod Craniofac Res 2015;18(3): 175–84.

38. Springer IN, Zernial O, Nolke F, et al. Gender and nasal shape: measures for rhinoplasty. Plast Reconstr Surg 2008;121(2):629–37.

39. Bass LS. Injectable filler techniques for facial rejuvenation, volumization, and augmentation. Facial Plastic Surgery Clinics of North America 2015; 23(4):479–88.

40. Rohrich R, Alleyne B, Novak M, et al. Nonsurgical rhinoplasty. Clin Plast Surg 2022;49(1):191–5.

41. Jasin ME. Nonsurgical rhinoplasty using dermal fillers. Facial plastic surgery clinics of North America 2013;21(2):241–52.

42. Kurkjian TJ, Ahmad J, Rohrich RJ. Soft-tissue fillers in rhinoplasty. Plast Reconstr Surg 2014;133(2): 121e–6e.

43. de Maio M. Ethnic and gender considerations in the use of facial injectables: male patients. Plast Reconstr Surg 2015;136(5 Suppl):40s–3s.

44. Petersen C, Markiewicz MR, Miloro M. Is augmentation required to correct malar deficiency with maxillary advancement? J Oral Maxillofac Surg 2018;76(6):1283–90.

45. Binder WJ, Azizzadeh B. Malar and submalar augmentation. Facial Plastic Surgery Clinics of North America 2008;16(1):11–32.

46. Akhavan AA, Ibelli T, Benaroch D, et al. Coverage gaps and inconsistencies: the landscape of insurance coverage for orthognathic surgery in the United States. FACE; 2023. https://doi.org/10. 1177/27325016231178338. 27325016231178338.

47. Nkenke E, Vairaktaris E, Kramer M, et al. Three-dimensional analysis of changes of the malar-midfacial region after LeFort I osteotomy and maxillary advancement. Oral Maxillofac Surg 2008;12(1):5–12.

48. San Miguel Moragas J, Van Cauteren W, Mommaerts MY. A systematic review on soft-to-hard tissue ratios in orthognathic surgery part I: maxillary repositioning osteotomy. J Cranio-Maxillo-Fac Surg 2014;42(7):1341–51.

49. Khamashta-Ledezma L, Naini FB. Prospective assessment of maxillary advancement effects: maxillary incisor exposure, and upper lip and nasal changes. Am J Orthod Dentofacial Orthop 2015; 147(4):454–64.

50. Chu YM, Bergeron L, Chen YR. Bimaxillary protrusion: an overview of the surgical-orthodontic treatment. Semin Plast Surg 2009;23(1):32–9.

51. Esenlik E, Kaya B, Gülsen A, et al. Evaluation of the nose profile after maxillary advancement with impaction surgeries. J Craniofac Surg 2011;22(6): 2072–9.

52. Hellak AF, Kirsten B, Schauseil M, et al. Influence of maxillary advancement surgery on skeletal and soft-tissue changes in the nose - a retrospective cone-beam computed tomography study. Head Face Med 2015;11:23.

53. Mommaerts MY. The ideal male jaw angle–An Internet survey. J Cranio-Maxillo-Fac Surg 2016; 44(4):381–91.

54. Gibelli D, Codari M, Rosati R, et al. A quantitative analysis of lip aesthetics: the influence of gender and aging. Aesthetic Plast Surg 2015;39(5): 771–6.

55. Stephen ID, McKeegan AM. Lip colour affects perceived sex typicality and attractiveness of human faces. Perception 2010;39(8):1104–10.

56. Rossi AM, Fitzgerald R, Humphrey S. Facial soft tissue augmentation in males: an anatomical and practical approach. Dermatol Surg 2017;43(Suppl 2):S131–9.

57. Kiessling P, Balakrishnan K, Fauer A, et al. Social perception of external laryngeal anatomy related to gender expression in a web-based survey. Laryngoscope 2022. https://doi.org/10.1002/lary.30498.

58. Glikson E, Sagiv D, Eyal A, et al. The anatomical evolution of the thyroid cartilage from childhood to adulthood: A computed tomography evaluation. Laryngoscope 2017;127(10):E354–8.

59. Dixson BJ, Sulikowski D, Gouda-Vossos A, et al. The masculinity paradox: facial masculinity and beardedness interact to determine women's ratings of men's facial attractiveness. J Evol Biol 2016;29(11):2311–20.

60. Epstein J. Facial hair restoration: hair transplantation to eyebrows, beard, sideburns, and eyelashes. Facial Plastic Surgery Clinics of North America 2013;21(3):457–67.

61. Shue S, Kurlander DE, Guyuron B. Fat injection: a systematic review of injection volumes by facial subunit. Aesthetic Plast Surg 2018;42(5): 1261–70.

62. Fedok FG, Mittelman H. Augmenting the prejowl: deciding between fat, fillers, and implants. Facial Plast Surg: FPS (Facial Plast Surg) 2016;32(5): 513–9.

63. Braz A, Humphrey S, Weinkle S, et al. Lower face: clinical anatomy and regional approaches with injectable fillers. Plast Reconstr Surg 2015;136(5 Suppl):235s–57s.

64. Rohrich RJ, Sorokin ES, Brown SA. In search of improved fat transfer viability: a quantitative analysis of the role of centrifugation and harvest site. Plast Reconstr Surg 2004;113(1):391–5. ; discussion 396-7.

65. Terino EO, Edwards MC. Customizing jawlines: the art of alloplastic premandible contouring. Facial Plastic Surgery Clinics of North America 2008; 16(1):99–122, vi.

66. Vargervik K, Ousterhout DK. Experiment augmentation of mandibular contour in gonial area. J Dent Res 1989;68.

67. Ousterhout D. Mandibular angle augmentation. In: Ousterhout D, editor. Aesthetic contouring of the craniofacial skeleton. Boston, MA: Little, Brown and Co; 1991. p. 431–40. chap 31.

68. Büttner M, Mommaerts MY. Contemporary aesthetic management strategies for deficient jaw angles. PMFA News 2015;2(4).

69. Sigaux N, Mojallal A, Breton P, et al. Mandibular Advancement Means Lower Facial Enlargement: A 2-Dimensional and 3-Dimensional Analysis. J Oral Maxillofac Surg 2018;76(12):2646.e1–8.

70. Choi TH, Kim SH, Yun PY, et al. Soft tissue changes after clockwise rotation of maxillo-mandibular complex in class III patients: three-dimensional stereophotogrammetric evaluation. J Craniofac Surg 2021;32(2):612–5.

71. Kwon JJ, Kang YH, Hwang DS. Delayed soft tissue changes after clockwise rotation of the maxillo-mandibular complex. J Craniofac Surg 2022; 33(7):2041–4.

72. Binder WJ, Dhir K, Joseph J. The role of fillers in facial implant surgery. Facial plastic surgery clinics of North America 2013;21(2):201–11.

73. Sykes JM, Fitzgerald R. Choosing the best procedure to augment the chin: is anything better than an implant? Facial Plast Surg 2016;32(5): 507–12.

74. Belmontesi M, Grover R, Verpaele A. Transdermal injection of Restylane SubQ for aesthetic contouring of the cheeks, chin, and mandible. Aesthetic Surg J 2006;26(1s):S28–34.

75. Sykes JM, Suarez GA. Chin advancement, augmentation, and reduction as adjuncts to rhinoplasty. Clin Plast Surg 2016;43(1):295–306.

76. Niamtu J. Lip reduction surgery (reduction cheiloplasty). Facial plastic surgery Clinics of North America 2010;18(1):79–97.

77. Sforza M, Andjelkov K, Zaccheddu R, et al. The "brazilian" bikini-shaped lip-reduction technique: new developments in cheiloplasty. Aesthetic Plast Surg 2012;36(4):827–31.

78. Claassen H, Mönig H, Sel S, et al. Androgen receptors and gender-specific distribution of alkaline phosphatase in human thyroid cartilage. Histochem Cell Biol 2006;126(3):381–8.

79. Deschamps-Braly JC, Sacher CL, Fick J, et al. First female-to-male facial confirmation surgery with description of a new procedure for masculinization of the thyroid cartilage (Adam's Apple). Plast Reconstr Surg 2017;139(4):883e–7e.

80. Irwig MS. Testosterone therapy for transgender men. Lancet Diabetes Endocrinol 2017;5(4):301–11.

81. Pang KC, Nguyen TP, Upreti R. Case report: successful use of minoxidil to promote facial hair growth in an adolescent transgender male. Front Endocrinol 2021;12:725269.

82. Epstein J, Bared A. Gender-affirming hair procedures. Operat Tech Otolaryngol Head Neck Surg 2023;34(1):19–29.

83. Unger RH. Female hair restoration. Facial Plastic Surgery Clinics of North America 2013;21(3):407–17.

84. Lv M, Yang X, Gvetadze SR, et al. Accurate reconstruction of bone defects in orbital-maxillary-zygomatic (OMZ) complex with polyetheretherketone (PEEK). J Plast Reconstr Aesthetic Surg 2022;75(5):1750–7.

85. Hussain RN, Clark M, Berry-Brincat A. The use of a polyetheretherketone (PEEK) implant to reconstruct the midface region. Ophthalmic Plast Reconstr Surg 2016;32(6):e151–3.

86. Narciso R, Basile E, Bottini DJ, et al. PEEK implants: an innovative solution for facial aesthetic surgery. Case Rep Surg 2021;2021:5518433.

87. Nocini R, D'Agostino A, Trevisiol L, et al. Mandibular recontouring with polyetheretherketone (PEEK) patient-specific implants. BMJ Case Rep 2022;15(4). https://doi.org/10.1136/bcr-2022-248826.

88. Scolozzi P, Martinez A, Jaques B. Complex orbito-fronto-temporal reconstruction using computer-designed peek implant. J Craniofac Surg 2007;18(1).

89. Ahmad AF, Yaakob H, Khalil A, et al. Evaluating patients' satisfaction level after using 3D printed PEEK facial implants in repairing maxillofacial deformities. Ann Med Surg (Lond) 2022;79:104095.

90. Rojas YA, Sinnott C, Colasante C, et al. Facial implants: controversies and criticism. a comprehensive review of the current literature. Plast Reconstr Surg 2018;142(4):991–9.

91. Khorasani M, Janbaz P, Rayati F. Maxillofacial reconstruction with Medpor porous polyethylene implant: a case series study. J Korean Assoc Oral Maxillofac Surg 2018;44(3):128–35.

92. Hashem FK, Al Homsi M, Mahasin ZZ, et al. Laryngotracheoplasty using the Medpor implant: an animal model. J Otolaryngol 2001;30(6):334–9.

93. Gafar Ahmed M, AlHammad ZA, Al-Jandan B, et al. Silicone facial implants, to fixate or not to fixate: a narrative review. Cureus 2023;15(2):e34524.

94. Kim IS. Augmentation rhinoplasty using silicone implants. Facial plastic surgery clinics of North America 2018;26(3):285–93.

95. Zaed I, Cardia A, Stefini R. From reparative surgery to regenerative surgery: state of the art of porous hydroxyapatite in cranioplasty. Int J Mol Sci 2022;23(10). https://doi.org/10.3390/ijms23105434.

96. Beirne OR, Curtis TA, Greenspan JS. Mandibular augmentation with hydroxyapatite. J Prosthet Dent 1986;55(3):362–7.

97. Maenhoudt W, Hallaert G, Kalala JP, et al. Hydroxyapatite cranioplasty: a retrospective evaluation of osteointegration in 17 cases. Acta Neurochir 2018;160(11):2117–24.

98. James SE, Herman JL, Rankin S, et al. The Report of the 2015 U.S. Transgender Survey. Washington, DC: National Center for Transgender Equality; 2016.

99. Moiduddin K, Mian SH, Umer U, et al. Design, analysis, and 3D printing of a patient-specific polyetheretherketone implant for the reconstruction of zygomatic deformities. Polymers 2023;15(4). https://doi.org/10.3390/polym15040886.

100. Wang Z, Yang Y. Application of 3D Printing in Implantable Medical Devices. BioMed Res Int 2021;2021:6653967.

101. Mian SH, Moiduddin K, Elseufy SM, et al. Adaptive Mechanism for Designing a Personalized Cranial Implant and Its 3D Printing Using PEEK. Polymers 2022;14(6). https://doi.org/10.3390/polym14061266.

102. Trinh LN, McGuigan KC, Gupta A. Delayed Granulomas as a Complication Secondary to Lip Augmentation with Dermal Fillers: A Systematic Review. Surg J (N Y) 2022;8(1):e69–79.

103. Sweis L, DeRoss L, Raman S, et al. Potential effects of repetitive panfacial filler injections on facelift surgery and surgical outcomes: survey results of the members of the aesthetic society. Aesthet Surg J Open Forum 2023;5:ojad010. https://doi.org/10.1093/asjof/ojad010.

104. Jacobsson J, Andreasson M, Kolby L, et al. Patients' Priorities Regarding Female-to-Male Gender Affirmation Surgery of the Genitalia-A Pilot Study of 47 Patients in Sweden. J Sex Med 2017;14(6):857–64.

105. Beek TF, Kreukels BP, Cohen-Kettenis PT, et al. Partial Treatment Requests and Underlying Motives of Applicants for Gender Affirming Interventions. J Sex Med 2015;12(11):2201–5.

106. Rohrich RJ, Bolden K. Ethnic rhinoplasty. Clin Plast Surg 2010;37(2):353–70.

107. Cobo R. Non-Caucasian Rhinoplasty. Clin Plast Surg 2022;49(1):149–60.

108. Heiman AJ, Nair L, Kanth A, et al. Defining regional variation in nasal anatomy to guide ethnic rhinoplasty: A systematic review. J Plast Reconstr Aesthetic Surg 2022;75(8):2784–95.

109. Cho DY, Massie JP, Morrison SD. Ethnic Considerations for Rhinoplasty in Facial Feminization. JAMA facial plastic surgery 2017;19(3):243.

110. Thomas M, D'Silva J. Ethnic rhinoplasty. Oral Maxillofac Surg Clin 2012;24(1):131–48.

111. Benjamin T, Knott PD, Seth R. Gender-affirming facial surgery: Anatomy and fundamentals of care. Operat Tech Otolaryngol Head Neck Surg 2023;34(1):3–13.

112. Olivieri P, Uribe FA, Quereshy FA. Aesthetic Facial Surgery and Orthodontics: Common Goals. Oral Maxillofac Surg Clin 2020;32(1):153–65.

113. Olivi P, Garcia C. Bi-maxillary advancement surgery: Technique, indications and results. Int Orthod 2014;12(2):200–12.

114. Singh S, Mehrotra D, Mohammad S. Profile changes after conventional and chin shield genioplasty. Journal of Oral Biology and Craniofacial Research 2014;4(2):70–5.

Facial Gender-Affirming Surgery
Pitfalls, Complications, and How to Avoid Them

Jacquelyn Knox, MD, William Y. Hoffman, MD*

KEYWORDS

- Facial feminization • Forehead contouring • Scalp advancement • Mentalis muscle

KEY POINTS

- It is critical to set expectations and understand the patient's goals for facial feminization.
- While component procedures of facial feminization surgery are common, specific complications and pitfalls can arise when combining these procedures toward the goal of feminizing the face.
- Understanding the patient's individual anatomy is essential for successful facial feminization surgery.

INTRODUCTION

Combining multiple technically challenging procedures into 1 larger operation, facial feminization surgery (FFS) provides many opportunities for both functional and aesthetic complications. Many of the component procedures such as rhinoplasty and genioplasty are common; however, special considerations arise both when performing these procedures in combination with one another and when applying them toward the specific goal of feminizing the face. In addition to the technical challenges of this operation, there are many challenges that stem from psychosocial issues experienced by patients seeking gender affirmation surgery. As such, thoughtful attention should be paid to patient selection, counseling, and expectation setting. While FFS is currently performed in a lower number of specialized centers, patient demand and accessibility continue to grow.[1] As surgeons from a variety of specialties, including otolaryngology and oral and maxillofacial surgery, begin to offer FFS, they are likely to encounter new challenges while performing these procedures for different aesthetic or reconstructive goals.[2] This article aims to provide a summary of common complications and pitfalls for select component procedures in FFS and share lessons learned in how to avoid them.

PATIENT COUNSELING AND EXPECTATION SETTING

During an initial consultation for FFS, it is important to assess the individual patient's goals. While some classically described features of a feminine face include a lower hairline, absence of frontal bossing, or a more obtuse nasolabial angle, most cis-gendered women do not have all these features. It is much more common to find "feminine faces" with some mixture of "feminine" features and some more "masculine" features. As such, we recommend starting any patient consultation with an open-ended question such as, "what bothers you the most?" This approach opens a dialog between the patient and surgeon, where both the patient's most important concerns are addressed while allowing the surgeon to use their expertise to make a comprehensive surgical plan.

Division of Plastic and Reconstructive Surgery, University of California San Francisco, 505 Parnassus, Suite M-593, San Francisco, CA 94143-0932, USA
* Corresponding author.
E-mail address: William.hoffman@ucsf.edu

Oral Maxillofacial Surg Clin N Am 36 (2024) 237–245
https://doi.org/10.1016/j.coms.2024.01.004

This open dialog about a patient's goals also provides a critical opportunity to set realistic expectations, both about the healing process and the final outcome. Many patients first experience gender dysphoria at a very young age and have faced significant psychosocial challenges related to gender dysphoria.[3] As such, these surgeries are highly anticipated, and patients often express desire for dramatic changes to their appearance or to be consistently recognized as a woman by others.[3] It is crucial to clearly convey the limitations of FFS; facial characteristics are just one part of what contributes to perceived "femininity," which also includes voice, manner of speech, movement, dress, and physical build, among other attributes. This senior author counsels every patient that when looking in the mirror after surgery, one will still recognize themselves; FFS cannot entirely change one's appearance but rather "softens" and "feminizes" the features. The healing process can also be challenging for patients who may expect more immediate results. Facial swelling, skin recoil, and scar maturation after FFS can take weeks to months. We find it helpful to take photos for tracking progress during the healing process. As with any surgery, it is important that the patient and surgeon have clear, open communication and that all goals are well aligned.

PITFALLS AND COMPLICATIONS BY FACIAL REGION

The following sections will focus on procedures within the upper, middle, and lower third of the face before commenting on some additional procedures this surgeon offers more frequently. While a brief description of each procedure will be included, details of surgical technique are beyond the scope of this article, which will focus primarily on pitfalls and complications. More common complications such as infection, hematoma, and seroma will not be addressed.

Upper Third

Consideration for procedures in the upper third of the face should start with a comprehensive analysis of the frontonasal-orbital region, including the nasofrontal angle, the contour of the frontal bone, the supraorbital ridge, the height of the forehead, the brow, and hairline shape.[4] Changes to the forehead and periorbital region can have a dramatic effect on one's appearance. Plain films of the face are ordered for all patients preoperatively to assess for the presence and extent of the frontal sinus (**Fig. 1**).

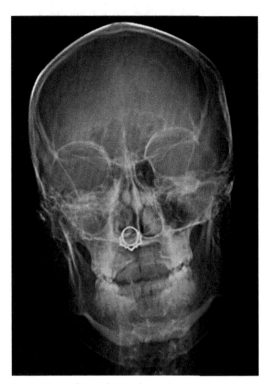

Fig. 1. Plain film of the face clearly showing the outline of the frontal sinus as well as the chin contour and gonial angles.

Hairline advancement and brow lift

This author most frequently performs hairline advancement in conjunction with brow lift using a pretrichial incision. A strip of scalp is removed, aiming for a length of approximately 55 to 60 mm between the medial brow and the hairline—the average length of a female forehead. If possible, without placing too much tension on the closure, more scalp can be removed from the temporal region where the hairline is often the most receded. If no hairline advancement is needed, a coronal incision can be used for brow lift with the advantage of a hidden scar. However, the position of the hairline must be carefully evaluated to avoid excessive elevation.

Pitfall: Unnatural appearing hairline or alopecia.

Cause: (1) Suboptimal incision design or placement, (2) damage to hair follicles, (3) flap ischemia.

Prevention: (1) If using a pretrichial incision, we have found that an irregular rather than straight-line incision along the hairline makes for a more aesthetic scar (**Fig. 2**). As with all coronal incisions (and the lateral extension of pretrichial incisions into the temporal hair-bearing scalp), the starting limb should be angled backward approximately 45° to camouflage the scar in the hair and avoid damage to facial nerve branches and the superficial temporal artery. (2) Galeal scoring to facilitate scalp

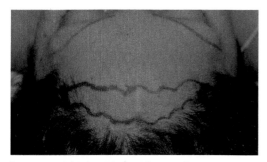

Fig. 2. Pretrichial incision with irregular pattern.

advancement and closure should be avoided as it does not greatly increase the amount of advancement possible and may cause additional ischemia of the scalp flap, leading to telogen effluvium. (3) This author uses Raney clips along the edges of the scalp flap for hemostasis. We recommend placing gauze sponges under the Raney clips to pad the skin and paying attention to how long they remain in place to avoid flap ischemia.

Pitfall: Inadequate hairline advancement.

Cause: (1) Failure to fixate the scalp under adequate tension. (2) Severity of androgenetic alopecia.

Prevention: (1) This author recommends setting adequate tension on the advanced scalp using a 2-0 polydioxanone suture looped around the plates used for frontal bone fixation and sutured to the galea posterior to the scalp incision (**Fig. 3**). If no osteotomy is performed, small drill holes can be placed in the supraorbital rim for this suture fixation. (2) In cases with significant temporal alopecia but more normal central hairline, temporal rotation flaps may be used to correct the hairline (**Fig. 4**). In cases of more severe hairline recession, adequate hairline advancement is not possible with standard techniques. In these cases, 1 option is staged hairline advancement

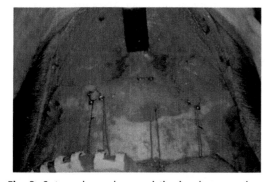

Fig. 3. Sutures looped around the hardware and sutured to the galea (not shown) to fix the scalp in an advanced position. Also note bone dust used to smooth contour irregularities and cover hardware.

starting with the placement of low-profile tissue expanders in the temporal regions followed by the advancement of expanded flaps at a second procedure.

Pitfall: Excessive hairline advancement.

Cause: Suboptimal incision selection and analysis of preoperative forehead length.

Prevention: This issue is rare. Most patients will benefit from hairline advancement as there is a high prevalence of androgenetic alopecia in this population and a feminine forehead is typically shorter in length. Coronal incisions for brow lift should thus be used sparingly in patients with shorter preoperative forehead lengths.

Forehead contouring

We most commonly utilize pretrichial or coronal incisions depending on the length of the forehead and position of the brow. Subgaleal dissection proceeds posteriorly to the level of the inferior nuchal line and anteriorly to the level of the zygomaticofrontal sutures to achieve adequate mobility of the scalp for closure. Care must be taken to avoid branches of the facial nerve in the temporoparietal region. A pericranial flap is carefully elevated from temporal line to temporal line, exposing the entire frontonasal-orbital region. For adequate exposure, dissection must proceed below the level of the supraorbital rim, exposing the zygomaticofrontal sutures laterally and the frontonasal suture medially. The supraorbital and supratrochlear neurovascular bundles must be protected during this process. In cases where there is no frontal sinus (5%–10%), contouring is performed solely with a burr. If frontal bone setback is required, osteotomies are planned by transilluminating the frontal sinus with a light cord (**Fig. 5**) and marking the borders with a sterile pencil. While virtual surgical planning is becoming increasingly popular for frontal sinus reconstruction, we find transillumination to be an effective, fast, and low-cost technique. Osteotomies to remove the anterior table are performed with a reciprocating saw (**Fig. 6**). After the anterior table is reshaped, it is fixated using low-profile titanium plates. Additional burring is necessary to smooth transitions and any contour irregularities.

Pitfall: Contour irregularities or palpable hardware.

Cause: Inadequate smoothing of the transition between the reconstructed anterior table of the frontal sinus and the native frontal bone.

Prevention: It is imperative to redrape the skin several times over the contoured frontal bone to check for the degree of correction and for any palpable irregularities before closure. Attention should be paid to the supraorbital rim where we

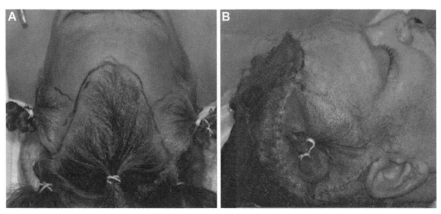

Fig. 4. (A) Preoperative markings in a patient with temporal alopecia. (B) Postoperative photo after temporal rotation.

find patients are more sensitive to contour irregularities. Additionally, bone dust which is gathered during the process of burring is used liberally to pack any irregularities, divots, and to cover any hardware (see **Fig. 3**). Avoiding injury to the pericranial flap during dissection is also helpful, as this provides additional soft tissue coverage over the reconstruction. The pericranial flap is closed carefully to avoid any visible or palpable step-offs in the forehead.

Pitfall: Temporal hollowing.

Cause: Ischemic injury, denervation, or disruption of the suspensory system of the temporal fat pad leading to fat pad atrophy[5]

Prevention: Some investigators have demonstrated lower rates of temporal hollowing using suprafascial dissection (above the superficial layer of the deep temporal fascia).[5,6] We essentially apply this technique, waiting until 1 to 2 cm above the level of the supraorbital rim to transition

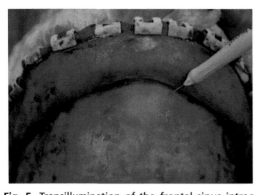

Fig. 5. Transillumination of the frontal sinus intraoperatively. This photograph shows the use of a small fiber which is placed through a drill hole; direct application of a reusable fiberoptic light to the surface of the bone works equally well.

through the superficial layer of the deep temporal fascia, staying above the fat pad, until reaching the lateral orbital rim.

Complication: Sinus dysfunction, sinus exposure, or mucocele formation.

Cause: Excessive shaving, poor osteotomy design, inadequate sealing of the sinus, or inadequate fixation[1]

Prevention: As described previously, preoperative imaging and intraoperative assessment with techniques such as transillumination of the sinus with a light cord are crucial in assessing for the presence and extent of the frontal sinus before performing any contouring or osteotomies. Additionally, patients should be assessed for history of frontal sinus disease, paying attention to history of frontal headaches or recurrent sinus infections. Preoperative ear, nose, and throat doctor referral should be considered for these patients, as they may be at higher risk for sinus dysfunction or mucocele.

Complication: Nerve injury.

Cause: (1) Injury to the supraorbital and supratrochlear nerves can occur when excess traction is placed on the bundles from failure to fully release them from the supraorbital notch of foramen (2) Injury to the frontal branch of the facial nerve can occur during coronal dissection.

Prevention: (1) It is important to differentiate whether the neurovascular bundles lay in a notch or foramen. If a foramen is present, we perform osteotomy using a mallet and osteotome. The bundles are then carefully released using a fine periosteal elevator and protected during contouring of the supraorbital rim using a malleable retractor. (2) This author prefers a deeper plane of dissection directly overlying the deep layer of the deep temporal fascia to minimize the risk of damage to the frontal branch of the facial nerve.

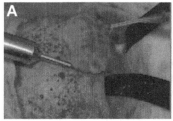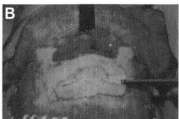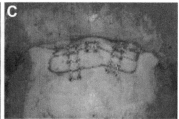

Fig. 6. (*A*) Frontal osteotomy with a reciprocating saw. (*B*) Completed frontal osteotomy. Pencil markings outline the high point of this piece of bone, where an additional osteotomy is performed to flatten the contour. (*C*) Contoured frontal bone fixated with hardware.

Complication: Diplopia.

Cause: (1) Trauma to the superior oblique muscle, tendon, or the trochlea itself. (2) Poor placement of osteotomy lines along the insertion of the trochlea on the orbital roof[7]

Prevention: (1) In the vast majority of cases, the trochlea will scar back into place without complication. However, this author has had 2 cases of persistent diplopia following contouring of the supraorbital region. We recommend limiting manipulation in the anterior orbit as much as possible to maintain the insertion of the trochlea. (2) The trochlea inserts onto the trochlear fovea, which is a slight depression on the anteromedial orbital surface.[8] As such, osteotomies should be planned carefully to avoid this region. In cases of persistent diplopia, consultation with ophthalmology is recommended.

Middle Third

A comprehensive evaluation of the middle third of the face includes the malar region, nose, nasofrontal junction, nasolabial junction, and upper lip. As the centerpiece of the face, the nose is particularly important to address and will often need global reduction in order to maintain balance with the rest of the feminized face.[9–11] In this author's experience, insurance coverage of feminizing rhinoplasty can be more challenging. We recommend careful documentation that addressing the upper and lower thirds of the face without adequately addressing the nose will significantly inhibit the overall goal of feminizing the face.

Rhinoplasty

The goals of a feminizing rhinoplasty are to reduce the overall size of the nose and to define and rotate the tip. Maneuvers to accomplish this goal will vary widely from patient to patient. For comprehensive rhinoplasty, this author most commonly performs open rhinoplasty using a stair-step incision across the columella and bilateral rim incisions. Dorsal hump reduction is performed with a rasp or osteotome. Cephalic trim and tip-defining sutures are routinely incorporated to reduce and refine the tip, accentuating the supratip break. To create a more obtuse nasolabial angle and prevent drooping of the tip, an anchoring suture is sometimes placed through the posterior aspect of the medial crura into the septum. To narrow the midvault, this author performs low-to-low osteotomies through less than 0.5 cm percutaneous incisions on the nasal sidewalls. Alar base and flare reduction is often necessary to achieve an overall narrower appearance.

Pitfall: Persistently masculine appearance despite global reduction of the nose.

Cause: Failure to address the nasofrontal transition.

Prevention: A more masculine appearance of the nasofrontal region is characterized by a more acute nasofrontal angle with prominent supraorbital rims and frontal bossing.[10,12] It is imperative that this area is addressed during forehead contouring to optimize the appearance of the nose after feminizing rhinoplasty. A radix graft, which this author makes with diced cartilage wrapped in a fascia, is often a useful adjunct in these circumstances.

Complication: Nasal obstruction.

Cause: Excessive narrowing of the midvault

Prevention: Significant narrowing of the midvault is often required, as masculine noses frequently have a wider bony base width.[11] Patients should be assessed preoperatively for other anatomic factors such as septal deviation and turbinate hypertrophy, which may increase the risk of nasal obstruction after feminizing rhinoplasty and should be addressed concurrently.[9] Dorsal hump reduction can also disrupt the integrity of the attachment between the septal dorsum and upper lateral cartilages, thereby collapsing the internal nasal valve. Spreader grafts may be necessary in these cases.[13]

Complication: Open roof deformity.

Cause: Over-resection of large dorsal hump.

Prevention: Over-resection of the dorsal hump can lead both to open roof deformity and distortion of the dorsal aesthetic lines. Osteotomies used to narrow the midvault should be fully mobilized, allowing medialization of the segments to assist in closing an open roof. Spreader grafts can be used as needed to restore the integrity of the dorsal aesthetic lines.[13]

Lip lift

This author performs lip lift with a typical "bullhorn" incision under the nasal sill. Skin incisions are carried down to the level of the orbicularis oris muscle, excess skin is removed, and the upper lip is undermined for 2 to 3 mm to allow tension-free closure.

Pitfall: Alar distortion, sill widening or deformation, and change in nostril shape.

Cause: Excess tension along the incision line, distortion of the anatomy of the nasal sill.

Prevention: When performing lip lift in conjunction with rhinoplasty, and particularly alar base reduction, it is important to carefully secure the new alar base within the alar crease. Excess tension on the incision line here can cause scar widening over time, leading to nostril and lip asymmetry.[9] Additionally, there are opposing forces at play between the downward tension on the lip lift incision and the desire for elevation of the nasal tip. As such, this author advises careful consideration before combining an upper lip lift with open rhinoplasty, and particularly alar base reduction. A lip lift can easily be staged as an office procedure under local anesthesia.

Pitfall: Disproportion of the lower third of the face.

Cause: Over-resection of the upper lip.

Prevention: While the extent of skin excision depends on the individual patient, in general a 3:1 ratio of philtrum to upper labial height is optimal. As recommended by Bluebond-Langner and colleagues,[14] no more than 25% of the original philtral height should be removed to avoid producing a "gummy" smile.[15]

Lower Third

The lower third of the face involves comprehensive examination of the jawline, including the gonial angles, width, height, and projection of the mandible. A more masculine chin is typically wider, taller, and has greater anterior projection with an overall "square" appearance.[16] Adequately addressing the overlying soft tissue is equally important as significant bony reduction and contouring.

Genioplasty

Genioplasty is performed using an intraoral incision between the canines, taking care to identify and protect the mental nerves bilaterally. While in some cases, adequate contouring can be achieved without osteotomy, most patients will require vertical or horizontal reduction. A 3-piece genioplasty is most commonly performed, utilizing 2 vertical osteotomies and 1 horizontal osteotomy to create a narrower and more pointed chin shape.[16] Osteotomies are performed in a standard fashion with a reciprocating saw. Bony segments are fixated in place using titanium plates and/or wires. The entire mandibular border is then contoured with a power rasp, taking care to smooth the transition between the native mandibular border and any fixated segments.

Pitfall: Persistently wide-appearing chin.

Cause: Failure to address or consider the soft tissue.

Prevention: Contouring the chin can be particularly challenging in higher body mass index (BMI), "full-faced," and older patients. In full-faced patients, even dramatic bony work may be obscured by overlying soft tissue fullness. In older patients, bony chin reduction may accentuate excess skin or skin laxity. We have found that plication of the mentalis muscle in the midline is extremely effective at narrowing the chin and perform this in almost every patient (**Fig. 7**). For higher BMI patients and older patients, it is important to counsel on the possible need for additional procedures such as liposuction, face lift, or neck lift to achieve optimal results.

Pitfall: Lip or chin ptosis/"Witch's chin"

Cause: Failure to resuspend the mentalis, or damage to the mentalis muscle.

Prevention: When making the intraoral incision, it is imperative to leave an adequate cuff of mentalis muscle for resuspension at the end of the procedure. If there is an inadequate cuff of muscle, absorbable sutures can be passed through the mentalis and suspended around the lower teeth to hold the muscle in place until adequate healing occurs.

Complication: Nerve injury.

Cause: Excess traction or sharp injury to the mental nerve.

Prevention: Temporary neuropraxia may occur from traction on the mental nerve, however permanent sensation loss is extremely rare. It is critical to have detailed knowledge of the course of the inferior alveolar and mental nerves. The mental nerve exits the mandible through the mental foramen, which can be found approximately at the level of the second premolar. Within the body of the mandible, this nerve takes a more inferior course before traveling superiorly to exit the bone, thus osteotomies should be performed at least 5 mm below the level of the mental foramen to avoid injury.[16] Additionally, this author utilizes a power

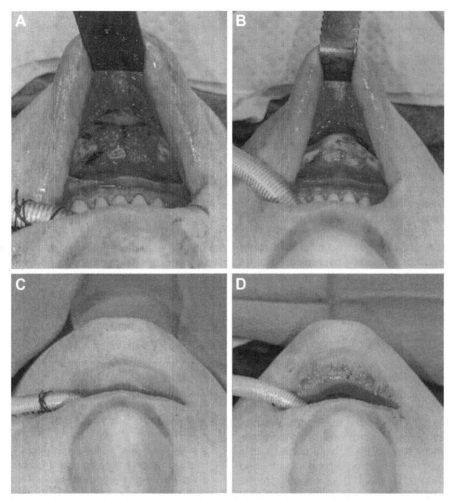

Fig. 7. (*A*) Intra-oral incision showing the mentalis muscle before plication. (*B*) Intra-oral incision showing the mentalis muscle after plication. Additionally, note significant contouring of the mandible. (*C*) External view of the chin before mentalis plication (but after mandible contouring). (*D*) External view of the chin after mentalis plication, showing obvious narrowing of the soft tissue of the chin.

rasp to contour the mandible rather than rotary instruments or power burrs, which are more likely to entrap neurovascular structures.

Gonial angle reduction

The gonial angles are accessed through lateral intraoral incisions, which can be performed as an extension of the midline incision or as 2 separate incisions. Dissection is performed carefully in a subperiosteal plan to fully expose the anterior, inferior, and posterior surfaces of the mandibular angle. Care should be taken to avoid injury to the retromandibular vein, which can cause bleeding that is difficult to control.

Pitfall: Persistently square-appearing jawline.

Cause: (1) Failure to adequately contour the body of the mandible. (2) Failure to address masseteric hypertrophy.

Prevention: (1) This author finds that a square-appearing mandible is often misattributed to the gonial angles. Contouring of the mandibular body and genioplasty produce far more dramatic changes to the overall appearance of the jaw than gonial angle reduction. However, gonial angle reduction can be useful in patients with excessive flaring of the angle, which can be assessed on physical examination and preoperative x-ray.[16,17] (2) A hypertrophic masseter can also contribute significantly to excess width in the lower third of the face. For these patients, we inject 50 units of botulinum toxin per masseter in multiple spots at the start of the procedure.

Other Procedures

There are several additional procedures that can be incorporated into facial feminization. We will discuss some of the more commonly used procedures at our institution.

Facial fat grafting

This author most commonly utilizes facial fat grafting to address areas including the malar region, tear troughs, and lips. The abdomen is an easily accessible donor site, and fat is harvested by hand using a 2.7-mm cannula with 10-cc syringes. This author uses a 22-gauge needle to make small stab incisions through which fat is injected with a 22-gauge blunt cannula.

Pitfall: Overcorretion or under-correction.

Cause: Unpredictability of fat resorption.

Prevention: This author does not recommend overcorrection, both because it is difficult to remove excess fat and because a "choke" effect has been described whereby over-injection of fat in a small space can precipitate fat necrosis.[18] Some amount of fat resorption is expected, and additional fat grafting can be easily performed in the office as needed.

Chondrolaryngoplasty or "tracheal shave"

Chondrolaryngoplasty addresses prominent thyroid cartilage, or "Adam's apple." This author uses a transverse submental incision, approximately 2 to 3 cm in length. The incision is carried through the subcutaneous tissue until the platysma is encountered, and then dissection proceeds inferiorly toward the thyroid cartilage in a preplatysmal plane. Blunt dissection is performed between the strap muscles. The pretracheal fascia and perichondrium are incised in the midline, and the perichondrium is elevated to expose the thyroid cartilage. The cartilage is reduced using a rongeur or power burr. The strap muscles and fascia should be reapproximated prior to skin closure.

Pitfall: Unesthetic scar.

Cause: Suboptimal incision placement.

Prevention: An unsightly scar is most common with a direct incision over the thyroid cartilage. Scars in this area can also become tethered to underlying structures, causing animation of the scar during speech or swallowing.[19] Some investigators recommend an intraoral approach, which typically requires additional equipment such as an endoscope.[20] This author prefers a submental incision, which is inconspicuous while allowing for adequate exposure with a lighted retractor.

Complication: Vocal complications.

Cause: Destabilization of the epiglottitis, injury to the vocal cords or laryngeal nerves during dissection[1]

Prevention: Thorough knowledge of anatomy is required to perform this procedure safely. The thyrohyoid membrane should not be violated during dissection along the superior border of the thyroid cartilage, as this places the superior laryngeal nerve at risk of injury. Minimal elevation should be performed on the internal surface of the superior thyroid notch to prevent disruption of the thyroepiglottic ligament and vocal cord attachments.[21] While this author has not found it necessary, direct visualization of the vocal cords via intraoperative endoscopy can be considered to minimize the risk of vocal complications.[19]

CLOSING THOUGHTS

While facial feminization is a technically challenging procedure with many potential pitfalls and complications, it is also extremely rewarding. Working with these patients is a privilege and has given this surgeon the opportunity to make significant improvements in overall wellbeing and quality of life for many transgender women.

CLINICS CARE POINTS

- Attention to detail including incision type, incision design, and smoothing contour irregularities is critical while addressing the upper third of the face.
- Preoperative plain films of the face and transillumination of the frontal sinus with a light cord intraoperatively are useful for assessing the presence and extent of the frontal sinus.
- Anchoring the hairline with sutures helps provide a reproducible result both for scalp advancement and brow lift.
- Failure to address the frontonasal region may lead to suboptimal results after feminizing rhinoplasty.
- Addressing the soft tissue with mentalis muscle plication in addition to bony mandible contouring is essential for addressing the lower third of the face.

DISCLOSURE

The authors have nothing to disclose.

REFERENCES

1. Simon D, Capitán L, Coon D, et al. Secondary Facial Gender Surgery: Causes of Poor Outcomes and Strategies for Avoidance and Correction. Plast Reconstr Surg 2023;347–57. https://doi.org/10.1097/prs.0000000000010324.

2. Cohen W, Maisner RS, Mansukhani PA, et al. Barriers To Finding A Gender Affirming Surgeon. Aesthetic Plast Surg 2020;44(6):2300–7.

3. Spiegel JH. Challenges in Care of the Transgender Patient Seeking Facial Feminization Surgery. Facial Plast Surg Clin North Am 2008;16(2):233–8.

4. Eisemann BS, Wilson SC, Ramly EP, et al. Technical Pearls in Frontal and Periorbital Bone Contouring in Gender-Affirmation Surgery. Plast Reconstr Surg 2020;326E–9E. https://doi.org/10.1097/PRS.0000000000007113.

5. Baek RM, Heo CY, Lee SW. Temporal dissection technique that prevents temporal hollowing in coronal approach. J Craniofac Surg 2009;20(3):748–51.

6. Matic DB, Kim S. Temporal hollowing following coronal incision: A prospective, randomized, controlled trial. Plast Reconstr Surg 2008;121(6):379–85.

7. Stallworth JY, Hoffman WY, Vagefi MR, et al. Superior oblique palsy after facial feminization surgery. Journal of AAPOS 2023;27(3):165–6.

8. Haug RH. Management of the trochlea of the superior oblique muscle in the repair of orbital roof trauma. J Oral Maxillofac Surg 2000;58(6):602–6.

9. Flaherty AJ, Stone AM, Teixeira JC, et al. Feminization Rhinoplasty. Facial Plast Surg Clin North Am 2023;31(3):407–17.

10. Di Maggio MR, Anchorena JN, Dobarro JC. Surgical management of the nose in relation with the fronto-orbital area to change and feminize the eyes' expression. J Craniofac Surg 2019;30(5):1376–9.

11. Rodriguez AM, Savetsky IL, Cohen JM, et al. Gender Considerations in Rhinoplasty. Plast Reconstr Surg 2023;438–45. https://doi.org/10.1097/prs.0000000000010159.

12. Bellinga RJ, Capitán L, Simon D, et al. Technical and clinical considerations for facial feminization surgery with rhinoplasty and related procedures. JAMA Facial Plast Surg 2017;19(3):175–81.

13. Teymoortash A, Fasunla JA, Sazgar AA. The value of spreader grafts in rhinoplasty: A critical review. Eur Arch Oto-Rhino-Laryngol 2012;269(5):1411–6.

14. Salibian AA, Bluebond-Langner R. Lip Lift. Facial Plast Surg Clin North Am 2019;27(2):261–6.

15. Dang BN, Hu AC, Bertrand AA, et al. Evaluation and treatment of facial feminization surgery: part II. lips, midface, mandible, chin, and laryngeal prominence. Arch Plast Surg 2022;49(1):5–11.

16. Wang MW, Rodman RE. Gender Facial Affirmation Surgery; Techniques for Feminizing the Chin. Facial Plast Surg Clin North Am 2023;31(3):419–31.

17. Simon D, Capitán L, Bailón C, et al. Facial Gender Confirmation Surgery: The Lower Jaw. Description of Surgical Techniques and Presentation of Results. Plast Reconstr Surg 2022;149(4):755E–66E.

18. Clauser L, Zavan B, Galiè M, et al. Autologous fat transfer for facial augmentation: Surgery and regeneration. J Craniofac Surg 2019;30(3):682–5.

19. Vandenberg KN, Plocienniczak MJ, Spiegel JH. Chondrolaryngoplasty. Facial Plast Surg Clin North Am 2023;31(3):355–61.

20. Shoffel-Havakuk H, Cohen O, Lahav Y, et al. Scarless Neck Feminization by Transoral Endoscopic Vestibular Approach Chondrolaryngoplasty: A Prospective Cohort. Otolaryngol Head Neck Surg 2023. https://doi.org/10.1002/ohn.296.

21. Sturm A, Chaiet SR. Chondrolaryngoplasty—Thyroid Cartilage Reduction. Facial Plast Surg Clin North Am 2019;27(2):267–72.

9780443128875